# STRENGTHENING VERSUS STABILISATION EXERCISE PROGRAMMES FOR PREVENTING AND REDUCING LOW BACK PAIN IN FEMALES

# STRENGTHENING VERSUS STABILISATION EXERCISE PROGRAMMES FOR PREVENTING AND REDUCING LOW BACK PAIN IN FEMALES

## QAIS GASIBAT

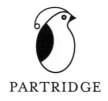

PARTRIDGE

ISBN:      Softcover            978-1-5437-4400-2
           eBook                978-1-5437-4401-9

**To order additional copies of this book, contact**
Toll Free 800 101 2657 (Singapore)
Toll Free 1 800 81 7340 (Malaysia)
orders.singapore@partridgepublishing.com

www.partridgepublishing.com/singapore

# CONTENTS

# LIST OF TABLES

# LIST OF FIGURES

# LIST OF ABBREVIATIONS

| | |
|---|---|
| sEMG | Surface Electromyography Activity |
| C1 | Cervical 1 |
| CLBP | Chronic Lower Back Pain |
| EMG | Electromyography |
| IOM | Establishment of Medication |
| LBP | Low Back Pain |
| NRC | National Exploration Committee |
| ONS | National Stats |
| SBTP | Stabilization Programme |
| SBTP | Stabilisation Training Programme |
| STTP | Strengthening Programme |
| UNISZA | Universiti Sultan Zainal Abidin |
| WHO | World Health Organisation |

# ABSTRACT

The prevalence of Low Back Pain (LBP) among women is disturbingly high due to the hormonal and reproductive factors such as irregular or prolonged menstrual cycle and hysterectomy. Physical therapists use a variety of exercises when treating patients with LBP. Hence, appropriate selection and designation of a training programme capable of stimulating the trunk and hip muscles would be beneficial in both rehabilitation and prevention of LBP. The current study compared the effectiveness of Strengthening Training Programme (STTP) with Stabilisation Training Programme (SBTP) intended to ascertain the most effective programme in stimulating the trunk and hip muscles. A total of 50 healthy females with normal BMI and ages ranging from 19 to 24 years were randomly allotted to STTP and SBTP. The participants underwent five different sets of exercise modalities for each programme three times a week for a period of five weeks. Electromyography (EMG) data were collected from five muscles of Rectus Abdominis, External Oblique, Multifidus, Gluteus Maximus, and Gluteus Medius. The readings from the EMG were compared at the initial phase and after the interventions using t-test. Both training programmes showed significantly increased in all of the muscle activities post-intervention. A statistically significant difference of post-intervention muscle activations between the two training programmes was also obtained ($p < 0.05$). The SBTP intervention was found to be more efficient in stimulating the back muscles activations as opposed to STTP. Therefore, stabilisation training programme could be a practical measure for prevention and rehabilitation of LBP among females.

# ACKNOWLEDGEMENTS

First, I would like to express my everlasting gratitude to Almighty God, our Creator, our Sustainer who has made it possible for me to complete this programme successfully and equally thank Him for His continued mercy and blessing. I would like to sincerely thank my main Supervisor Professor Dr Nordin bin Simbak and Co-supervisor Dr Aniza Abd Aziz for their constructive comments, valuable suggestions and good guidance. I equally thank them for their kindness and necessary encouragement. I am extremely indebted to them, as I have learnt so much from them.

I am profoundly grateful to Ministry of Higher Education and Scientific Research, Libya for supporting me throughout my education in all possible ways and for providing a haven when I need them the most.

My sincere appreciation goes to my mother, and of course, my wife and my kids. I am also grateful to my brothers and sisters for their love, patience, moral support, encouragement and concern throughout my studies. Thank you all for having faith in me, and I am glad we can all share in this success. I love you all.

My appreciation goes to some of my colleagues during the programme and all my friends and colleagues at Home.

# CHAPTER 1

## INTRODUCTION

## 1.1 Background of the Study

Low Back Pain (LBP) is among the most prevalent health issues in various communities worldwide, particularly in industrialised nations. About 80% of people living in these countries are affected by LBP, at least for a period of time during their life (Reid, 2004; Damasceno et al., 2006). Furthermore, LBP is currently a notable injury in Asian societies with a rate of 8.5% (Chaiamnuay et al., 1998; Khan, 2014). It is categorised as Chronic Low Back Pain (CLBP) when it lasts longer than three months and as acute LBP when it lasts for less than 12 weeks. Meanwhile, sub-acute LBP lasts from six to 12 weeks (Beinart et al., 2013; Karşılaştırılması, 2014; Watson et al., 2002).

Around 15% to 45% of the world's population suffers from CLBP (Karunanayake et al., 2013). LBP is the number one cause of activity limitation and absence from work worldwide. It also causes a huge financial burden on individuals, family members, communities, industries, and government authorities (Nachemson et al., 2000; Metgud et al., 2008; Hoy et al., 2010; Karunanayake et al., 2013). There has been much research in Europe on evaluating the interpersonal, economic effect of LBP. In Europe, LBP continued to be the most prevalent cause of disability among young adults, with over 100 million working days lost each year (Sozen, 2010).

A survey carried out in Sweden found that work-time lost due to LBP increased from seven million in 1980 to 28 million in 1987 (Centre for Disease Control and Prevention, 2001; Duthey, 2013). In the US, LBP ranked the second most common cause of disability in grown-ups and one of the significant reasons for working days lost. It has been estimated that 149 million times of work are dropped annually due to LBP (Guo et al., 1999; Stewart et al., 2003; Ricci et al., 2006; Katz, 2006). LBP incurs a very high economic cost, estimated at between US$100 and US$200 billion per year, two-thirds of which are because of reduced wages and lost productivity (Carey et al. 1996; Rubin, 2007).

Different factors cause back pain including ageing, smoking, chronic stress, nutrition disorders, and hereditary reasons, weight gain, and incorrect lifting of heavy dumbbells (Mannion et al., 1999; Ogawa et al., 2005). It is assumed that decreased back muscle endurance causes muscle fatigue and overloads smooth tissue and passive constructions of the lumbar spine, leading to LBP (Marras et al., 1987; Wilder et al., 1996). Muscle weakness is usually associated with LBP. Also, changes in the size of back lordosis have for long been speculated to be the main reason for LBP (Williams, 1955; McKenzie & May 1981).

Experts have recently examined the significance of certain trunk, hip, muscle strengthening, and stabilising training to prevent injuries (Baratta et al., 1988; Leetun et al., 2004). Weakness and poor stamina of the lumbar and gluteus muscles have also been observed in individuals with lower extremity of accidental injuries and LBP (Biering-sØrensen, 1984; Kankaanpää et al., 1998; Leinonen et al., 2000; Nourbakhsh & Arab, 2002; Leetun et al., 2004). In this regard, discovered that athletes with no history of injury had stronger muscles.

Reduced flexibility, lowered disk liquid, and in other words, the indigent physical conditions of individuals, almost all decrease the efficacy of disk placed in the spinal cord (Mannion et al., 1999). Based on this idea, reducing the trunk muscle's mass endurance leads to muscle exhaustion and adds pressure around the soft tissues and non-active structures of the spine (Ebrahimi et al., 2005). Furthermore, since the endurance capacity of muscle tissue provides an indication of muscle fatigue, there is a belief that people with less strong muscles in the trunk area are more likely to experience strength pressures, which may cause high pressure on the spine, leading to CLBP (Lee et al., 1999; Ebrahimi et al., 2005).

Increased body mass index and decreased muscle strength have also been found to be directly associated with persistent LBP while obesity and reduced trunk muscle power are significant factors in long-term LBP, and as such, a trunk muscle strengthening system will be beneficial in easing the pain (Bayramoglu et al., 2001). Muscle strength and tiredness limit the patient's physical functioning (Pedersen & Saltin, 2006).

Numerous treatment strategies such as joint mobilisation and manipulation, soft tissue massage treatment, electrotherapy, acupuncture, and traction are used in clinical practice for the treatment of LBP with different degrees of efficacy. Treatment simply by improving the coordination, versatility, stabilisation, endurance, and power of muscle through appropriate exercises will restore the total amount and proper function of muscles (Ebrahimi et al., 2014).

Physiotherapists commonly prescribe exercises for CLBP, as a supportive intervention. The popularity of exercising in LBP treatment continues to grow. It has been traditionally used particularly in sports activities performance and rehabilitation (Sozen, 2010). It is also possible to use exercise as a physical or behavioural tool to enhance physical function, lower the intensity of back pain and also to decrease back pain-related impairment (Rainville et al., 2004).

Furthermore, findings from systematic reviews indicated the effectiveness of exercise in managing CLBP (Hides, Jull, & Richardson, 2001; Hayden et al., 2005; Lewis et al., 2008). The conclusion from the majority of the studies showed that active exercises are a therapeutically desirable approach in managing LBP, although there is no general agreement on the best types of exercise, intensity or active intervention (Abenhaim et al., 2000). Exercise therapy seems to be the most frequently applied physical therapy in individuals with back pain (Bouchard et al., 1990). It eliminates pain, improves and maintain the whole range of motion, the vigour and strength of lumbar and abdominal muscles, thus facilitating early restoration of normal function (Cady et al., 1979; Bouchard et al., 1990).

The use of mechanical support to the lower back contributes to recovery with least likelihood of relapse. Workout training is frequently employed to improve function in LBP rehabilitation and to avoid deconditioning of lumbar musculature and persistent LBP. Research established that exercise reduces pain, invigorate muscle tissue, lower mechanical stress to spinal structures, enhance level of fitness, prevent injury, and boost posture and mobility in patients with LBP (Cady et al., 1979; Jackson & Brown, 1983; Shiple & DiNubile, 1997; Chok et al., 1999; França et al., 2010).

Several studies suggested that exercise highly effective for the treatment of LBP. Exercise not only facilitate functional enhancement but also lower the pain and considerably improve the vigour and endurance of the patient (Lee et al., 2008; Ebrahimi et al., 2014). Exercise is the most commonly used intervention to optimise recovery from LBP. In effect, exercise can minimise the frequency and severity of relapses (Macedo et al., 2013).

In summary, exercise therapy has been successfully used to restore chronic and recurrent LBP, quite certainly in short-term rehabilitation (Hayden et al., 2005; Helmholtz et al., 2008).

## 1.2 Statement of the Problem

It is evident from the literature that females have significantly higher LBP problems than males (Pavón, 2016). This is logical as most of the studies in this area showed that females reported more LBP issues than males. However, according to the Spain national survey conducted in 2006, which focused on health issues in this regard, there was 19.9% prevalence of LBP among females during the year. It has been established that reproductive factors are related to CLBP especially in females. These factors include unbalanced, persistent cycle and hysterectomy (Wijnhoven et al., 2006; Pavón, 2016)

To the best of the researcher's knowledge, there is not a single study that concentrated on determining the best and most effective modality exercises for reducing LBP in females. Many previous studies compared various exercise modalities for reducing LBP. Some of these studies recommended McKenzie (Machado et al., 2006; Garcia, 2013), while others suggested yoga exercise (Sherman et al., 2005; John et al., 2007; Tekur, 2008; Sherman et al., 2011). Also, a study conducted by Hosseinifar et al. (2013) suggested stabilisation exercise. However, the majority of the studies found no difference between the exercise modalities for reducing LBP (Petersen et al., 2002; Danneels et al., 2001; Slade & Keating, 2006). There has been no clear evidence that one of the exercise programmes is superior to another in reducing LBP. Therefore, a wide range of exercises have been used for progressive strengthening of the back and hip muscles (Faas, 1996; Van et al. 1997).

## 1.3 Rationale for the Study

LBP clinical guidelines recommend staying active and earlier return to normal activity as the way to more rapid restoration with less likelihood for disability and fewer recurring problems (Waddell et al., 1997; Royal College of General Practitioners, 1999; Abenhaim et al., 2000). Increasing back strength may also result in an effective therapeutic intervention intended for LBP.

Stabilisation and strengthening exercise strategies are believed to be capable of increasing the trunk area and back strength. Also, individually designed exercise programmes appeared to be effective. Strengthening and neuromuscular rehabilitation of the core musculature can be beneficial in restabilising the spinal column and in turn minimise instability-related pain (Kibler et al., 2006). The main focus of core strengthening is to stabilise the abdominal, paraspinal and gluteal musculature. The most significant types of exercise for preventing LBP include those related to abdominal muscles, dorsal muscles and gluteal muscles (Nadler, et al., 2002).

However, there is absolutely no clear evidence that one type of exercise is more effective than another in non-specific LBP. Every modality involves specific motions for specific muscles. The preferred exercises are those deemed simpler to be performed and more beneficial for people with back pain. They can decrease the likelihood of future back injuries, thereby preventing work absenteeism. A regular mixture of exercises also results in quicker return to work, less persistent disability and fewer recurrence problems (Waddell et al., 1997).

**Electromyography** (EMG) offers a way to analyse the activation levels of the back muscles while exercising (Arokoski et al., 2001; Davidson & Hubley-Kozey, 2005; Ekstrom et al., 2007; Stevens et al., 2007). The findings of this research could be beneficial for physiotherapists in deciding the specific mode of exercise and site of muscles when treating and monitoring the progress of patients with LBP from low-intensity exercises to those that need more muscle activities. These exercises would be useful for a core rehabilitation or performance improvement programme, based on the individual requirements of a patient or athlete.

## 1.4 Research Questions

1. Does strengthening exercise programme improve the trunk and hip muscle activities in females?

2. Does stabilisation exercise improve the trunk and hip muscle activities in females?

3. Are there significant differences between strengthening and stabilisation exercise programmes in the improvement of the trunk and hip muscle activities in females?

## 1.5 General Objective

This study aims to compare the effect of the strengthening and stabilisation type of exercise programmes on the trunk and hip muscle activities in females.

## 1.6 Specific Objectives

1.  To compare the EMG muscle activities of pre- and post-strengthening exercise programme on the trunk and hip muscles in females.

2.  To compare the EMG muscle activities of pre- and post-stabilisation exercise programme on the trunk and hip muscles in females.

3.  To compare the EMG muscle activities between strengthening and stabilisation exercise programmes on the trunk and hip muscles in females.

## 1.7 Operational Definitions

1.  Back muscle strength is contributed by the trunk and hip/lower limb muscles.

2.  Trunk muscles in this study comprised of three muscles; rectus abdominal, external oblique, and multifidus muscles.

3.  Hip or lower limb muscles in this study comprised of two muscles; gluteal maximus and medius muscles.

4.  Muscle activation was measured by Surface Electromyography activity (sEMG).

## 1.8 Hypotheses

1.  Strengthening exercise programme improves the trunk and hip muscle activities in females.

2.  Stabilisation exercise programme improves the trunk and hip muscle activities in females.

3.  There are significant differences between strengthening and stabilisation exercise programmes in the improvement of the trunk and hip muscle activities in females.

## 2.1 Low Back Pain

LBP is a pain restricted to the lumbar region extending from the second-level rib enclosure to the waistline (twelfth thoracic/first lumbar to fifth lumbar/first sacral vertebrae) and frequently incorporates transmitting leg pain, for example, sciatica. It is frequently marked as 'a non-particular' by the National Establishment for Wellbeing and Clinical importance (Savigny et al., 2009) because of its strain and soreness, and it is impractical to distinguish a particular reason for the pain. It has been estimated that in 85% of LBP cases, a non-particular pathoanatomical determination can be found (White III & Gordon, 1982; All Nachemson, Waddell, & Norlund, 2000). Non-particular LBP is additionally classified as acute, sub-acute or chronic. Acute pain happens abruptly and keeps going less than 6 weeks. Sub-acute pain lasts between 6 and 12 weeks, though the pain grows continuously. Whereas, chronic pain lasts more than 12 weeks and is recurrent (Frymoyer, 1988).

The 'regular history' of LBP is depicted as the lion's share of LBP and acute LBP cases recouping before chronicity, and the tremendous expenses related to LBP are because of those with persistent LBP (Savigny et al., 2009). In this manner, CLBP is looked upon by some as an extraordinary element from LBP and intense LBP (Bayramoglu et al., 2001). In any case, while there is an assortment of further co-morbidities related to, and which create incessant LBP, for example, psycho-social variables, it ought to be noted that coherently all CLBP invariably begins as acute LBP (Adams, Stefanakis, & Dolan, 2010). In fact, rather than the regular idea of LBP's normal history, including recuperation of most acute LBP, there is an evidence that a significant amount (69% to 75%) of low back damage and acute LBP develops into persistent LBP (Croft, Macfarlane, Papageorgiou, Thomas, & Silman, 1998), frequently with expanding recurrence and severity (Donelson, McIntosh, & Hall, 2012).

CLBP is a multifactorial condition with a wide assortment of related physical dysfunctions, including but not restricted to constrained scope of lumbar movement (Langevin & Sherman, 2007) and irregular stride (Lamoth et al., 2002; Anders et al., 2005; Langevin & Sherman, 2007; Lamoth, Stins, Pont, Kerckhoff, & Beek, 2008; Shambrook et al., 2011). The National Exploration Committee (NRC) and The Establishment of Medication (IOM) master boards recognise this and the multifactorial idea of a musculoskeletal issue in the populace as a whole (Waddell & Burton, 2001). Recently, various models attempting to explain, predict, and coordinate the multifactorial idea of LBP have been published (Waddell & Burton, 2001; Paul W Langevin & Sherman, 2007; Richmond, 2012; Hodges & Smeets, 2015). Despite the fact that a range of symptoms and dysfunctions may be observed in persistent LBP, it is not clear whether they are directly responsible for the pain experienced, but there is possible pain causing systems that may be identified with these dysfunctions. LBP continues to be a very common and expensive condition, even though much work has been done to investigate its causal factors and prescribed medication.

## 2.2 Prevalence, Costs, and Impact of LBP

In the United Kingdom, direct health care costs of LBP were £1632 million in 1998 (Maniadakis & Gray, 2000). There is a related economic loss due to the cost of informal treatment and productivity losses (Smith, 1999). Annually in the UK, up to 55 million working days are dropped due to LBP (Waddell & Burton, 2001). As such, it is estimated that the total economic cost of LBP ranges from £5 billion to £10 billion (Smith, 1999; Maniadakis & Gray, 2000). Nearly all these on-going costs originate from CLBP sufferers (Council, 2001). These costs are common among the majority of the traditional western industrialised countries (Smith, 1999). A cost of illness research regarding LBP in the Netherlands in 1991 found that the total costs were 0.28% to 1.7% of Gross National Item (Steenstra et al., 2006). This amounted to USD$4.6 billion, of which 93% were for indirect costs (absenteeism and disablement). Regarding function losses, LBP emerged as the costliest disease category. The total economic costs during 2001 in Sweden was approximately $86 billion, with 84% resulting from indirect costs (Ekman, Johnell, & Lidgren, 2005). During the 1980s, billions of dollars were annually estimated in the US (Pollock et al., 1989).

It is estimated that 149 million working days are lost annually because of LBP (Guo anise que al., 1999), which (if indirect costs from the UK and Sweden are comparable) would represent a massive indirect cost to the US economy. Total costs to the US economy have been recently approximated as USD$100-USD$200 billion annually (Katz, 2006). Freburger et al. (2009) also indicated that the number of people using public medical health insurance (i.e. Medicare and Medicaid) had increased substantially, suggesting that the bulk of increased direct costs from health care utilisation has already been supported through tax-financed systems. Although different health insurance and social care systems are not directly comparable (Dagenais, Caro, & Haldeman, 2008), it is clear that the prevalence of LBP is, in reality, a major contributor to the costs borne by the health solutions in developed western communities.

Common treatments used for LBP contribute to the high direct LBP-associated expenses (Katz, 2006). For instance, Katz (2006) emphasised that Doctor and Physician appointments are projected to be very expensive - £100 each and increasing to £6000 for medical check-ups. Surgery costs will be considerably higher, ranging from £21,000 to £55,500, but surgery can often be averted using more cost-effective treatments. Van Tulder, Koes, and Bouter (1995) estimated that total direct medical costs of treatment constituted $367 million, of which US$200 million was for medical centre care costs. This is probably because of the higher costs of hospital care (USD$3,856 to USD$5,782 per inpatient). Even though outpatient care is comparatively less expensive (USD$199 to USD$298; per outpatient), the higher rates of LBP incidence mean this adds up substantially to the total costs.

Based on the Office of National Stats (ONS) Omnibus Survey (presented in the Social Trends report), 40% of adults in the UK had experienced back pain lasting for more than one day in the last 12 months (Walker & Cooper, 2000). Evidence of prevalence is varying at a given point in time and the wide range of figures from studies has been attributed to the absence of uniform strategies (12% to 33% of point frequency, 22% to 65% for occurrence, and 11% to 84% for lifetime prevalence (Walker, 2000). More recently, it has been suggested that one-third of the UK population are affected annually (Walker & Cooper, 2000). Waddell and Burton, (2001) calculated that 60% to 80 % of adults would experience LBP at some point in their life. Andersson, Chaffin, and Pope (1991) provided several studies demonstrating even higher rates of LBP prevalence, including persistent and recurrent LBP.

The results reported by Freburger et al. (2009) showed that the US prevalence levels of LBP might have increased slightly (6%). It is unclear if this is a true reflection of increased prevalence of LBP, or perhaps due to decreased willingness to tolerate (Walker, 2000). It is not easy to confirm possible explanations through observation of prevalence, even though the ONS Health of Adult, The UK survey, whilst echoing the increased sickness and invalidity benefit claims, provided data indicating that there was hardly any change in the frequency between 1971 and 1981 (Walker, 2000).

Even though different studies have been using different approaches, it is obvious that LBP is highly common (and has been so for a while) and is expensive in developed western populations. The World Health Organisation (WHO) similarly reported rates of back pain disorders as being very high worldwide and as a cause of morbidity (Group, 1998).

In fact, non-westernised indigenous people have been found to suffer relatively high rates of LBP, including Australian Aborigines (Honeyman & Jacobs, 1996; The Steering Committee for the Review of Government Service Supply, 2007; Barrero et al., 2006). It is astonishing that there is a substantial prevalence of LBP in indigenous populations, yet rates of other so-called 'diseases of civilisation' such as weight problems, cancer, heart disease, type 2 diabetes (which have not risen drastically in occurrence over the last half-century among western populations) will be almost non-existent if they should stick to traditional diet and lifestyles (Andersson, 1999; Lindeberg, Cordain, & Eaton, 2003; Carrera-Bastos, Fontes-Villalba, O'Keefe, Lindeberg, & Cordain, 2011).

## 2.3 The Implications of LBP

Despite the difficulty of determining its accurate prevalence, most studies highlighted LBP as an issue of increasing concern across a wide range of populations. The personal burden and economic costs associated with such rates of prevalence are obvious. Therefore, understanding the LBP aetiology and determining effective interventions is essential in reducing this problem.

The increasing level of incapacity caused by LBP has huge financial ramifications (Troup, 1996). There is lack of effort to develop evidence-based practice approaches for the treatment of LBP. Although it is widely acknowledged that acute LBP has a short, common history and ought to be a favourable, self-constraining condition, the big issue related to the highest recurrent rate is frequently ignored (Waddell, Somerville, Henderson, & Newton, 1992). With one-year recurrent rates evaluated between 20% and 86% (Bergquist-Ullman & Larsson, 1977; Troup, 1996), the need to address this issue is imperative (Moffett, Richardson, Sheldon, & Maynard, 1995). There has been a global consideration for the restorative expenses related to LBP, which has certainly prompted a noticeable increase in the number and extent of studies in this direction.

## 2.4 Incidence and Prevalence of LBP

Information from epidemiological examinations in different countries show that lifetime incidence of LBP ranges from 49% to 70%, point predominance ranges from 12% to 30% and period pervasiveness ranges from 25% to 42% (Van et al., 2000). About 90% of people with LBP quit counselling with their doctor within three months (Croft et al., 1998), which is the most widely-recognised reason for limited action in individuals below 45 years old (Andersson et al., 1991).

Although LBP frequency increases in both childhood and adulthood, there are indications that lifetime prevalence is as high as 70% to 80% among 20-year-olds (Taimela, Kujala, Salminen, & Viljanen, 1997). Furthermore, a few studies have confirmed new initial rates of around 20% over a one to two-year time span. Point predominance increases with age, and it is higher in young women than in young men (Watson et al., 2003). Although numerous teenagers report certain impediments in daily exercise, for most of them, LBP is non-specific and self-constraining (Patton, 2015). Despite the fact that back pain is by all accounts a typical element in both men and women, the related spinal weaknesses and handicaps are more typical in women (Andersson, 1999).

An epidemiological investigation in the Netherlands examined a random sample of 161 general specialists from 1987 to 1988, utilising the Worldwide Order of Essential Care, the rate of LBP was particularly higher among women than among men and the frequency was highest for individuals between 25 and 46 years old. In the USA, back pain percentage has a yearly frequency of 10% to 15% and a point pervasiveness of 15% to 30% among the grown-up population (Van Tulder, Furlan, Bombardier, Bouter, & Group, 2003). The pervasiveness increases with age up to 65 years (Wilke, Wolf, Claes, Arand, & Wiesend, 1995). However, the results of most investigations on the occurrence and regularity of LBP differ significantly, depending on the participants' age and methodological differences. There is confusion that results from the use of various terms for LBP which all mean the same thing, such as non-particular LBP, lumbago, mechanical LBP, and idiopathic LBP (van der Velde & Mierau, 2000).

## 2.5 Risk Factors of LBP

Cigarette smoking, alcohol drinking and insufficient exercise have been proposed as risk factors in LBP (Deyo & Bass, 1989). Cigarette smoking could interfere with the blood circulation to the intervertebral disk, structures and nerve roots, leaving them more vulnerable to damage (Holm & Nachemson, 1988). There is proof that people who drink alcohol exhibit more episodes of back pain than teetotallers (Turk, Meichenbaum, & Genest, 1983). Likewise, fire-fighters who are unfit experience more episodes of back pain than those who are fit (Deyo & Bass, 1989). However, these are likely the lifestyle elements that are simply part of other possible trigger factors.

Two work-related issues are part of trigger factors of LBP: exposure to oscillation (Andersson et al., 1991) and heavy lifting (Kelsey et al., 1984). Knowledge of risk factors may help prevent back pain. Although the best goal should be to prevent LBP, the reality of this is doubtful given that LBP is a common occurrence (Waddell, Feder, & Lewis, 1997). In the meantime, it is essential to determine the potential of chronic groups at the earliest possible time and offer an adequate rehabilitation programme before disability becomes an issue.

## 2.6 Diagnosis of LBP

There have been numerous proposed causes of LBP over the years. These include disk degeneration, lumbosacral strain, sacroiliac disorders, joint aspect disorders, fibrositis, myofascial syndrome, and coccydynia. However, there is no medical evidence for any of these causes becoming the cause of LBP. The danger is that the patient will probably be given a nominal analysis, which is just a convenient packaging to put on the symptoms. It leads the patients to believe they may have degenerated, arthritis, or slipped disk and makes them dread the worst (Deyo, 1996).

## 2.7 The Nature of Back Pain

Pain has been depicted as a stand-out among the problems that must be addressed (Turk et al., 1983). Most patients who visit physiotherapy divisions have a complaint of pain. Pain differs in intense, period and significance. Relieving pain has brought about extraordinary medications in the past, such as rankling, dying, measuring, cutting, cleansing, harming and no less unusual medicines in the present, such as warming, solidifying, needling and transcutaneous nerve increase (Turk et al., 1983).

The subjective experience of pain is too high to escape from a reason or to look for a relief. This desire can make pain an effective factor in the sufferer's life, creating fear of any conduct that causes pain. The global relationship for the Investigation of Pain defines pain as "a disagreeable, tangible and passionate experience related to real or potential tissues, harm, or depicted as far as such" (Martin, Church, Thompson, Earnest, & Blair, 2009). Pain is experienced only by the individual (Moffett et al., 1995). The main way clinicians can increase their comprehension of pain is by getting pain reports from the patient.

## 2.8 The Relationship between Physical Activity and LBP

The value of physical exercise has been accepted as a major strategy in universal guidelines for those involved in the management of severe and CLBP (Arnau et al., 2006; Van Tulder et al., 2006). The advice to stay active, take early and gradual steps in the introduction of exercise, avoid bed rest are among the significant guidelines for primary care in LBP management (Koes, van Tulder, Ostelo, Burton, & Waddell, 2001; Bekkering et al., 2003). On the other hand, effective ways of managing LBP and avoiding recurrences and chronic situation can be elusive (Kent & Keating, 2008; Refshauge & Maher, 2006), and there is an urgent need to develop approaches for the prevention of CLBP (Majid & Truumees, 2008).

The possible role of physical activity in preventing CLBP has been proposed (Karmisholt & Gotzsche, 2005). Recently, it has been found that the advice to stay active has been recognised as a key aspect of active self-management of CLBP (Liddle, Gracey, & Baxter, 2007). Although studies have investigated activity programmes as a management strategy for severe and CLBP (Hendrick et al., 2011; Steenstra et al., 2006), such studies failed to evaluate activity levels in free-living, and as such, there is no possibility of identifying the relationship between any change in activity and its impact on LBP recovery. Currently, LBP patients have been advised to maintain, restore, and even increase their activity level as part of their general administration (Hendrick et al., 2011).

## 2.9 Muscle Weakness and LBP

Professionals have recently examined the level of specific trunk, hip, and muscle tissue strengthening for the prevention of injuries (Biering-sØrensen, 1984; Baratta et al., 1988). Some weaknesses and poor stamina from the lumbar and gluteus muscle tissues have also been observed in people suffering from lower extremity injuries and LBP (Biering-sØrensen, 1984; Baratta et al., 1988; Leinonen, Kankaanpää, Airaksinen, & Hänninen, 2000; Nourbakhsh & Arab, 2002).

Spine stability is provided by the bone, disk, ligaments, and muscle support. Segmental insufficient stability of the lumbar backbone could be responsible for functional disorder, stress and pain (Grieve, 1982; Stokes & Frymoyer, 1987). Paravertebral and abdominal muscles can be very efficient in improving the stability of the spine. Paravertebral and stomach muscles are also moderating factors of discomfort (Richardson & Jull, 1995; Paul W Hodges & Richardson, 1999).

Weakened abdominal muscles have been found to be a factor leading to LBP in people with CLBP, and during pregnancy for women, the abdominal muscles are overstretched and may be weak (Fast, Weiss, Ducommun, Medina, & Butler, 1990). Also, there is evidence of the relationship between poor trunk muscle tissue function and LBP (Lee et al., 1999). Individual abdominis has been recognised to play a role in separate aspects of spinal control (Cresswell, Oddsson, & Thorstensson, 1994; Hodges & Richardson, 1997; Paul W Hodges & Richardson, 1999; Arab & Ebrahimi, 2005). For instance, the rectus abdominis, internus obliquus, and externus obliquus are involved in direction-specific patterns regarding limb activity, hence providing postural support for leg movement (Cresswell et al., 1994). Subsequently, these muscle tissues are connected to manage trunk steadiness and motions of the vertebrae.

The rectus abdominis originates from the pubic crest and pubic symphysis and inserts at the cartilage of the 5th to seventh ribs and xiphoid process (Tortora & Grabowski, 2003). When contracted, the rectus abdominis flexes the vertebral line and compresses the stomach (Tortora & Grabowski, 2003). The rectus abdominis is believed to possess a high recruitment threshold, which can be significant in supporting the spine for high-load actions such as when pushing and lifting heavy objects (Jenkins & Tortora, 2011). According to Moore, Dalley and Agur (2013), the rectus abdominis is mainly activated in traditional and abdominal exercises and helps in increasing spinal movements (Moore et al., 2013).

External oblique originates from the lateral surface of the 5th to 12th ribs, the lower 8 ribs and inserts at the iliac crest (Moore et al., 2013). The lateral fibres of the external oblique compress the belly and flex the vertebral column

(Moore et al., 2013). Once there is a unilateral contraction of the external oblique, the vertebral column is laterally flexed and rotated (Moore et al., 2013).

Numerous investigations have demonstrated that multifidus is the central muscle in lumbar segmental stability, using its location within the posterior sacrum and iliac. In fact, it is inserted in the spinous procedure for the backbone except the cervical 1 (C1), and this muscle mass activates lateral flexion and trunk extension (Moore et al., 2013).

The gluteal muscles are a group of three muscles which make up the buttocks the gluteus maximus, gluteus medius and gluteus minimus. The three muscles originate from the ilium and sacrum and insert on the femur. The functions of the muscles include extension, abduction, external rotation and internal rotation of the hip joint (Moore et al., 2013).

## 2.10 The Benefit of Exercise and its Relationship with Reduced Pain in LBP

The ability of exercise to avoid and reduce LBP involves muscle physiology. Lowered intramuscular density in CLBP patients is usually due to atrophy of muscle mass fibres supplementary to disuse or very long loop response inhibition of back musculature (Arokoski et al., 1999). Moreover, deconditioned muscles possess a lowered ability to face trouble and repeated load, resulting in strain within the annular materials of the back disk and possibly leading to back pain (Reiman et al., 2009)

Also, there is a close association between back pain and muscles. Hip-extensor strength and hip-adductor endurance might lead to discomfort in the lumbar region (Reiman, Weisbach, & Glynn, 2009). Hip abductor weakness is typical in patients with LBP (wk Lee & Kim, 2015). People who mention LBP have come across a decrease in muscle mass electric power, muscle endurance, adaptability, and limitation of back as well as lower limb joint flexibility (Mannion, Adams, Cooper, & Dolan, 1999).

Those who suffer from LBP often try to avoid experiencing painful movements and eventually reduce activity resulting in the gluteus maximus and lowered muscle endurance (Smith, 1999). Gluteus maximus has also been found to cause fatigue quicker in individuals with LBP (Kankaanpää, Taimela, Laaksonen, Hänninen, & Airaksinen, 1998). Also, avoidance of annoying movements of the pathological backbone leads to the subsequent reconditioning from the back and hip muscle tissue. The finding is connected to improved fatigue levels coming from gluteus maximus and highlights the necessity to include this muscle in LBP rehabilitation to minimise the cycle concerning pain prevention behaviour (Reiman et al., 2009).

Elevated hip strength leads to minimising pain and advancements in function. With exercise treatment programmes for LBP people, adding popular muscle fitness exercise that may include back pain exercise will be ideal for rehabilitation and maintenance of smooth daily routine (Lewis, Morris, & Walsh, 2008).

Many studies have suggested that long-term research should show solid proof about exercise as a great intervention for LBP and recommended physical exercise for the management of severe LBP and CLBP (Chou et al., 2007; Chou & Huffman, 2007; Lewis et al., 2008). In this regard, Leetun, Ireland, Willson, Ballantyne, and Davis (2004) found that sports athletes who had not been injured had more powerful muscles.

The lumbar multifidus muscle is believed to be especially required in stabilising. Multifidus has been recognised to be atrophied in several reports by infiltration of fats in patients with long-term LBP (Danneels et al., 2001; Barker, Shamley, & Jackson, 2004; Leetun et al., 2004).

The pain causes atrophy of the paraspinal, isolated multifidus, quadratus lumbar, psoas, and gluteus maximus muscles in varying degrees, most significantly in the multifidus (Arokoski et al., 1999; Kamaz, Kiresi, Oguz, Emlik, & Levendoglu, 2007). The multifidus is the most medial from the lumbar back muscles, and is shown to be of greater importance than the longissimus thoracic and ilicostalis lumborum muscles in stabilising the lumbar spine (Arokoski et al., 1999; Kamaz et al., 2007; Cooper et al., 2013; wk Lee & Kim, 2015).

Reduced flexibility, less drinking water, and poor physical status of individuals invariably lower the efficiency of the disk in the spinal cord (Mannion et al., 1999). By this idea, reduced trunk muscle tissues endurance results in muscle exhaustion and heightened pressure through the soft tissues and non-active structures of the spine (Lee et al., 1999). Moreover, as the muscle tissue endurance capacity is a measure of muscles fatigue, it is believed that individuals with significantly less muscular strength in the trunk area muscles are definitely more vulnerable to strength pressures, which might trigger improper pressure around the backbone and aggravate CLBP (Cresswell et al., 1994; P W Hodges & Richardson, 1997).

Increased body mass index and decreased muscle strength were discovered to be directly associated with persistent LBP. Similarly, obesity and reduced trunk area muscle power are significant factors in persistent LBP. Trunk area muscle mass strengthening system will probably be effective in reducing the discomfort (Hodges & Richardson, 1999). Muscle power and fatigue limit the individual's physical functioning (Hodges & Richardson, 1998). Numerous intervention approaches, including joint mobilisation and treatment, soft tissue massage techniques, electrotherapy, and acupuncture have been employed in clinical practice for the treatment of LBP with varying degrees of success.

Physiotherapists prescribe exercises for LBP, but only as a supporting intervention for CLBP patients. Furthermore, results from the literature review indicate that exercise is effective in the treatment of CLBP (Oddsson, 1988; Hodges & Richardson, 1999). Many investigations have concluded that active exercises are an effective therapeutic strategy in managing LBP, regardless of the lack of agreement on the ideal approaches and level of the exercise (Arab & Ebrahimi, 2005).

Exercise therapy appears to be one of the most commonly applied physical therapy strategies for individuals with back pain (Bayramoglu et al., 2001). The general objective of this therapy strategy is to abolish discomfort, fix and maintain the maximum range of motion, improve the skills and endurance of the back and abdominis, thus adding to the timely restoration of regular function (Bayramoglu et al., 2001; Hayden, Van Tulder, Malmivaara, & Koes, 2005).

Towards this end, mechanised support for the lower back, which is usually helpful for recovery with least likelihood of relapse, is normally provided. Exercise is typically used to increase function in LBP rehabilitation and stop deconditioning of the back musculature to avoid persistent LBP (Abenhaim et al., 2000; Lewis et al., 2008). It is believed that exercise will positively reduce soreness, strengthen muscle tissue, lower physical stress to vertebral constructions, improve levels of fitness, prevent injury, and boost placement and mobility in people with LBP (Cady, Bischoff, O'connell, Thomas, & Allan, 1979).

## 2.11 Treatment of LBP: Staying Active

Medical guidelines recommend that health professionals should not advise or use bed rest as a treatment for LBP patients at a severe level. This recommendation is based on the result of the systematic reviews of literature associated with bed rest (Van Hall, Raaymakers, Saris, & Wagenmakers,

1995; Waddell et al., 1997). The results of these systematic reviews concluded that bed rest compared to staying active has no effect, but could prove slightly dangerous cases of acute non-specific LBP.

Clinical guidelines for staying active suggest advising patients to stay as active as possible, to continue regular daily activities, to stay at work or perhaps return to work as soon as possible, and gradually increase physical activities for more than a few days or a week. Systematic reviews by Bigos et al. (1994) and Waddell et al. (1997) reported faster rates of restoration, less pain and less impairment in back pain patients who were advised to stay active compared to individuals with no guidance. The reports of these researchers also indicated that suggestions to stay active led to much less sick leave and persistent disability compared to medical administration.

## 2.12 Treatment of LBP: Physiotherapy and Exercise

Physiotherapy is often used in the treatment of LBP, with an estimated 9% of patients with back pain going to physiotherapists (Maniadakis & Gray, 2000). Notwithstanding, there is still little conclusive evidence supporting any specific physiotherapeutic treatment of acute or repeated LBP (Evans & Richards, 1996). The economic burden caused by LBP in Britain has indicated the need to provide efficient, cost-effective therapy as a research priority. An estimated £36 million was spent on therapy by both the UK public and private sectors in the year 1992/1993 (Moffett et al., 1995). More recently, a comprehensive analysis of the economic consequence of LBP in the UK estimated that out of 1632 million immediate health care expenses, 37% were associated with physiotherapy and care coming from allied specialists (Maniadakis & Gray, 2000).

The scope of physiotherapy in LBP encompasses many prevalent treatment modalities that can be commonly split into 'passive' modalities including warmth, mobilisation and manipulation, therapeutic massage, traction and electrotherapy and 'active' modalities such as workout regimes and education (Foster, Thompson, Baxter, & Allen, 1999). The passive treatment modalities of mobilisation and manipulation (often termed as 'manual therapy') encompass some different methods such as stabilisation exercises and many others, such as stretching and yoga exercises (Kaltenborn, 1970; McKenzie & May 1981; Maitland, 2005).

Physiotherapists play a key role in conveying beneficial advice and treatment to patients with back pain. On the other hand, there is an evidence of disagreement about the efficacy of physiotherapy interventions. Some studies recognised certain specific exercise programmes for acute LBP to be ineffective (Malmivaara et al., 1995) while others have proved that some specific exercise programmes have been able to reduce the recurrences of LBP in comparison with general exercise programmes (Halldin, Zoega, Kärrholm, Lind, & Nyberg, 2005). There is an evidence that basic exercise programme is beneficial in building people's confidence and ability make use of their spine naturally (Halldin et al., 2005).

It is a common belief that Physical Activity plays a crucial role in the treatment of patients with LBP (Alaranta et al., 1994; Bendix, Bendix, Haestrup, & Busch, 1998; Halldin et al., 2005; Hicks, Fritz, Delitto, & McGill, 2005; Hurwitz, Morgenstern, & Chiao, 2005). In recent times, there have been many reports on the efficacy of specific exercise programmes, particularly spinal stabilisation exercise treatments in the management of acute and CLBP.

A serious problem for LBP sufferers is the considerably restricted range of movement of the trunk and pelvis. One of the most observable benefits of exercise is the ability to enhance or preserve musculoskeletal and cardiovascular function (Rainville et al., 2004). Exercise-based spine rehabilitation programmes are typically designed based on relieving discomfort, reinforcing the back, improving back flexibility, and improving functional activities and basic wellness. Research findings showed that damage to trunk area (Hurwitz et al., 2005), versatility (Waddell et al., 1997) and stamina (van der Velde & Mierau, 2000) were found in many people with CLBP. There is a convincing proof that exercise as part of comprehensive treatment increases quality of life, health, and significantly reduces sick leave (Bendix, Bendix, Labriola, Hæstrup, & Ebbehøj, 2000; Edmonds, McGuire, & Price, 2004; Kool et al., 2004; Storro, Moen, & Svebak, 2004; Pedersen & Saltin, 2006; May et al., 2008; Martin et al., 2009).

Successful training interventions will probably have a positive effect on general health and functional capacity (Pedersen & Saltin, 2006). Activities of everyday living like physical work can be performed in a lower percentage of maximum capacity and improve the standard of living (Martin et al., 2009). A large number of researchers have suggested that future investigations should reveal a strong proof with regard to exercise as a great intervention regarding LBP and recommend physical activity in the management of acute and CLBP (Cooper et al., 2013; Chou et al., 2007; Martin et al., 2009; Reiman et al., 2009). In this regard, Leetun et al. (2004) found that athletes who were not injured had stronger muscles.

It is believed that reducing trunk muscle tissue endurance contributes to muscle fatigue and increases pressure throughout the soft cells and non-active structures of the spine (Abenhaim et al., 2000) Likewise, since the muscle tissues endurance capability is an indication of muscle fatigue, it is believed that individuals with less muscle strength in trunk region are more vulnerable to power pressures (Bayramoglu et al., 2001; Lewis et al., 2008).

Exercise is continuously gaining popularity in LBP treatment. It has been traditionally used, especially in the fields of sports activities and rehabilitation (Sozen, 2010). Exercise can be used as a physical or perhaps behavioural device to enhance physical function and lessen back pain (Abenhaim et al., 2000).

Treatment simply by improving the dexterity, versatility, stabilisation, endurance, and power of muscle through appropriate exercise will restore the amount and function of muscles (Lee et al., 1999). Much research has suggested that exercise as a treatment of LBP works better than the common treatments. Exercise not only enhances the function of muscles but also decrease the pain and considerably raises the electric power and endurance of the individual (Lee et al., 1999; Mannion et al., 1999). Exercise is one of the most reliable treatments of LBP. In fact, it is effective in lowering the number and severity of recurrences (Holmes et al., 1996)

In summary, exercise therapy is a highly effective method for relieving CLBP and persistent LBP, at least in the short-term intervention (Mannion et al., 1999). On the other hand, extensive research typically shows specific treatments of different exercise strategies, including aerobic exercises, strength and stamina reconditioning and mobilising exercises (Cresswell et al., 1994; Mannion et al., 1999).

## 2.13 Types of Exercise Programme for LBP

Many detailed exercise applications have been suggested to enhance spinal stability (Parnianpour, Nordin, Kahanovitz, & Frankel, 1988). Specific exercises have already been suggested to activate muscle tissue (Arokoski et al., 1999; Morais, 2011). Exercise program in the management of LBP has been the subject of many systematic reviews that have produced varying results [(Richardson & Jull, 1995). The relative value of aerobic training (Moffett et al., 1995) and classified activity programmes, including McKenzie therapy (McKenzie & May 1981) and spinal stabilisation training (Richardson & Jull, 1995) are central to much of the debate.

Evidence for the use of exercise in LBP has further been supported by recent international comparison of medical guidelines for the management of LBP (Bayramoglu et al., 2001). Even though most of the guidelines do not usually extend recommendation beyond the acute stages, some of them (Netherlands, Philippines, Denmark and the UK) recommended exercise as an essential intervention with no regularity regarding the type and strength of the exercise. The significance of using exercise in the management of LBP is accordingly clear. However, the exact nature of the exercise remains vague.

Some studies have shown that the trunk muscles of individuals with CLBP are weaker compared with those of healthy individuals, and many programmes endorsed the use of strengthening training to rectify this disability (Arab & Ebrahimi, 2005). Strengthening training is the most studied type of training used to develop the lumbar strength (Rainville et al., 2004). Several authors recommended different conditions of strengthening training.

Certain resistance exercises apply specially designed equipment (Holmes et al., 1996). Some propose weight training, utilising body weight as a level of resistance, which includes simple floor exercises, the use of an exercise ball or perhaps techniques. In this kind of exercise, the lower section of the body is fixed on a system or table and the remaining part of the body is lifted or perhaps suspended from the edge of the platform using trunk muscles (Macedo, Bostick, & Maher, 2013). A review of 23 papers (Koes, Bouter, & van der Heijden, 1995) also suggested that part of specific back exercises was inconclusive. Various types of specific exercise management, such as Williams flexion exercises and McKenzie extension exercises, have been advocated for treating LBP during the past few years, with each advocate claiming that his/her exercise is the best, thus making the whole issue contradictory and confusing.

A study found no significant difference between flexion and extendable exercises (Hintermeister, Lange, Schultheis, Bey, & Hawkins, 1998). Different prominent authors in the field claim that theoretical evidence is growing in preference of an active exercise approach instead of any specific exercise (Waddell & Burton, 2001).

Randomised restricted trials of an intensive programme, guided by objective measurement using isokinetic start strength measurements, have reported extremely good results (Mayer et al., 1985) in a trial of patients with chronic mid back pain. They reported that 87% of the treatment group go back to work in comparison with 40% of the controls. Hazard et al. (1989) replicated the system and reported an identical 81 % and 40% return to work for the two teams respectively.

Rehabilitation programmes have reported benefits from some exercises. Kellett, Kellett, and Nordholm (1991) reported less back pain and less absence from work after exercise intended for an hour three times a week. Research in British (Ferreira, Oliveira, Ribeiro, Tafuri, & Vitor, 2006) randomly allocated individuals with CLBP into a fitness programme and a control group. Both groups were taught home exercises. The treatment group likewise attended eight exercise classes over a four-week period. This group showed a substantial improvement in disability, discomfort, and went for walks of distances longer than the control group. The authors concluded that the programme would be easy to operate and would not require any expensive equipment.

Research has indicated that neuromuscular dysfunction and tiredness of the back and abdominal muscles are prevalent amongst patients with back pain (Richardson & Jull, 1995). A recent development in the different treatment modalities of LBP has proposed substantial training of the trunk muscles, known as specific segmental stabilisation training or muscle disproportion techniques. Moreover, a primary clinical study has shown that early treatment of this dysfunction helps the LBP patients with instability and acute back pain to fully recover (Hides et al., 2001). However, despite the favourable preliminary results, the effect of incorporating these exercises for the treatment purposes and in a population with recurrent LBP has not been broadly researched.

## 2.14 Stabilisation Programme (SBTP) and Strengthening Programme (STTP) for LBP

Stabilisation Training Programme (SBTP) has become the most well-known treatment method for spinal rehabilitation due to the efficacy it has demonstrated in alleviating–discomfort and disability related to the spine. However, a few studies have reported that specific exercise programme reduces soreness and disability in persistent but not in acute LBP, although it can be helpful in remedying the acute LBP by minimising recurrence rate (Fahey, Insel, & Roth, 2012).

SBTP for individuals with LBP has evolved. Recently, there has been a focus on exercises that aim to maintain stability in the lumbar spine (Richardson & Jull, 1995). This type of exercise approach continues to be termed as lumbar stabilisation, primary stabilisation, or segmental stabilisation. Although there is no formal meaning of SBTP, this approach is usually aimed at improving the neuromuscular control, strength, and stamina of muscles central to maintaining dynamic spinal and trunk stability. Several categories of muscles are targeted, especially lumbar multifidus and other paraspinal, abdominal, diaphragmatic, and pelvic muscles. Standaert, Weinstein, and Rumpeltes (2008) reported that with the widespread clinical use of SBTP, it is necessary to critically assess the evidence for their efficacy in patients with CLBP. To this effect, SBTP has become an important conceptual and medical consideration in the management of patients with CLBP in the last 15 years. The overview of the available evidence shows that SBTP is effective in improving pain and function in a heterogeneous group of patients with CLBP. Moreover, through evidence-based criteria, there is certainly moderate evidence that SBTP is effective in improving discomfort and dysfunction in a heterogeneous number of patients with CLBP (M. Van Tulder et al., 2003).

In another perspective, Strengthening Training Programme (STTP) is defined as the built-in result of several force-producing muscle tissues performing maximally, either isometrically or dynamically during a solitary voluntary effort of a described task (Hoff & Helgerud, 2004). Power is a product of force and the ability to create as much force as possible in a shortest possible time (Hoff & Helgerud, 2004).

As with aerobic training, muscular strength advancements vary inversely on procession with initial training position. A muscle strengthens when it is extended close to its current pressure generating capacity. To improve maximal strength, psychological evidence revealed that training for 2 to 3 days a week, applying major muscle groups. Another study has also reported that STTP could increase muscle tissue which is beneficial, especially for individuals with long-term atrophy through the use of usually 8-12 repetitions (Tesch & Larsson, 1982).

## 2.15 Electromyography Measure of Muscle Activities

Electromyography (EMG) studies help researchers in understanding issues or problems related to the motion system. The problem may be localised towards the peripheral nervous system, or maybe the muscle itself and sometimes can be at the neuromuscular junction. This kind of diagnostic tool is precious in the differentiation and diagnosis of nerve and muscle mass diseases (Cresswell et al., 1994).

EMG is also used in the morphological evaluation of the motor unit (Katirji, 2007). It is important to synchronise the systems that supply motion picture data with EMG to look for the period when different muscle tissues join the muscle movements. These systems use digital cameras, electrodes and other relevant equipment to deliver information about the position, speed and acceleration measurements.

EMG is the electrodiagnostic study of muscles and nerves which can be applied in two distinct test components: Lack of conduction studies and EMG. Nerve bail studies measure how well and how fast the nerve fibres can send electrical indicators (Morgan, 1989). Lack of conduction studies can be explained as the recording of a peripheral nerve organs at some location far away from the site where a propagating action potential is caused by a peripheral nerve (Garcia & Vieira, 2011). Nerve conduction research provides unique quantitative details about neurological function in individuals with a variety of neuromuscular disorders (Clarys, Scafoglieri, Tresignie, Reilly, & Van Roy, 2010). The utilisation of muscles in the right and economical fashion helps increase activity and prevents injury. The most important points to accomplish healthy training are the follow-up of progress and carrying out corrections where necessary (Beck et al., 2009; Hendrix et al., 2009). EMG analysis can determine muscle tissue activation and fatigue and helps achieve the development of overall performance (Balestra et al., 2001). EMG in current sports studies also deals with determination and descriptions of the muscle types (Merletti, Rainoldi, & Farina, 2001).

The EMG testing involves evaluation of the electrical activity of a muscle mass and is one of the fundamental areas of the electrodiagnostic medical assessment. It is both an art and a science. It requires a comprehensive knowledge of anatomy in the muscles being tested, equipment settings and neurophysiology in the fine (Weiss et al., 2010). Morgan (1989) revealed that acquiring the information produced by active muscle mass provides knowledge about the activities of motor control centres. This can be accomplished invasively by wires or perhaps needles inserted directly into the muscle, or by placing electrodes over the surface of the skin overlying the investigated muscle tissue.

EMG recordings are performed with intramuscular needle electrodes. Nevertheless, surface electrodes are used in the study of sports technology. Most of the issues affecting this kind of modality have already been covered.

Electrodes are almost always sited along the physique of the muscle in question, with locations one-third and two-thirds along the length being standard. As mentioned earlier, small pre-amplifiers are often used in order to increase signal-to-noise ratios, especially seeing that telemetry of signals is increasingly used in order to preserve ecologically valid movement habits (Morgan, 1989; De Luca,1997; Hintermeister et al., 1998;Andersen et al., 2010; Clarys et al., 2010;). Once the signal is filtered and amplified, some types of rectification of the signal are applied.

Another evidence has also demonstrated that EMG is commonly used to measure the degree of muscle activation and provide a rough estimate of workout intensity for specific muscle tissue involved in the movement (Andersen et al., 2010). EMG signal has its contributions to finding the human body muscle mass functions (Illyés & Kiss, 2005). According to Ekstrom, Donatelli, and Carp (2007), EMG is the recording of the electric activity of muscles and comprises an extension of the physical search and testing of the motor system's honesty. EMG analysis can offer information related to the relative amount of muscular activity a workout requires and the optimal placement for the exercise (Basmajian & De Luca, 1985). Electro-physiological methods enable us to easily obtain useful information about neuro muscular activity (Massó et al., 2010).

## 2.16 Surface Electromyography

Surface Electromyography (sEMG) is a non-invasive way of measuring electrical muscle activity that occurs during muscle compression and relaxation cycles. sEMG is unique in revealing what a muscle does during movement and postures. Moreover, it objectively discloses the fine interaction or coordination of muscle tissue (Massó et al., 2010). sEMG is widely used in many applications, such as medical, practical neurology, gait and posture analysis, urology (treatment of incontinence), psychophysiology rehabilitation, physical therapy, physical and neurological rehabilitation, active teaching therapy in ergonomics, product certification of sport activities, biomechanics, movement analysis, athletes strengthening training and sport treatment and motion analysis (Cram, 1998; Bogey, Cerny, & Mohammed, 2003; Fauth et al., 2010).

sEMG refers to EMG and steps of muscle activity in microvolts. This form of feedback permits us to determine if muscles are not involved in a particular ability required to be calm, or involved in an ability needed to discharge the correct sequence with the right vigour. In addition to using sEMG feedback for training reasons, the information can also provide insight into the athlete's strength and fitness or the effects of an injury rehabilitation programme (Baars et al., 2007). sEMG can also be used to examine the service characteristics of specific muscles. Amplitude and power range of sEMG are commonly utilised to quantify neuromuscular activity and fatigue (Vinjamuri, Mao, Sclabassi, & Sun, 2006).

Even though the non-invasive nature of sEMG makes this technique ideal for medical use and research, sEMG data can be variable, which usually raises questions about the reliability of this technique (Bogey et al., 2003). Repeatability of sEMG data is established for many isometric exercises, sEMG which is sometimes called kinesiological EMG, is the EMG evaluation that makes it possible to obtain the signal from a muscle mass in a moving body (Cram, 1998). It should be noted that by using clarification, its use is restricted to actions that require a dynamic movement. sEMG is usually used to indicate which muscles are active. Surface electrodes are often attached to the muscle groups to be studied.

Clarys et al. (2010) explained that there are over 600 skeletal muscle tissues in the human body, and the two irregular and complex involvements of the muscles may result from neuromuscular diseases and intentional occupational or sports motions. Sports movement techniques and skills, training approaches and methods, and ergonomic verification of the human-machine interaction possess have a highly specialised muscle activity in common. The sources of sEMG signal muscle tissues produce electrical potentials because of action potentials. With electrodes placed on the surface or in muscle tissues, muscle action possibilities can be determined. Several events need to occur before contraction of muscle fibres. Central nervous system activity initiates a depolarisation in the motor neuron (Zipp, 1982; Lamontagne, 2002). Depolarisation is usually conducted along the motor neuron towards the muscle fibre's motor endplate. At the endplate, a chemical substance is released. This substance diffuses across the synaptic space and causes a depolarisation of the synaptic membrane. This trend is called muscle action potential. The depolarisation of the membrane layer spreads along the muscle materials, producing a depolarisation wave which can be detected by recording electrodes (Zipp, 1982).

The knowledge of such muscular action in its aspects, its evaluation and feedback should allow for the promotion of movement, sport components, training possibilities, and sport performance (Micheli, 2010). Some researchers argued that for example, concluding 32 sports, making over 100 different organic skills, including methodological EMG study, are an impossible job. EMG and sports are a vast area, and the entire coverage of such studies is almost impossible because information will be found spread in different journals, including those on the aspects of sports, ergonomics, biomechanics, and applied physiology in various congress procedures (Micheli, 2010).

Specifically, sEMG is a crucial tool of biomechanical research (De Luca, 1997; Soderberg & Knutson, 2000). It has also contributed to identifying the role of the muscles in some specific activities (Majid & Truumees, 2008). The sEMG has increasing importance in sports and work-related medicine and ergonomic research (Potvin & Bent, 1997; Balestra, Frassinelli, Knaflitz, & Molinari, 2001). It may also establish dynamic analysis, and for that reason, it is important in sports (Clarys, 2000; MacIsaac, Parker, & Scott, 2001).

## 2.17 Examples of Current sEMG Studies in Sports Sciences

sEMG has been a subject of lab research for decades. Only recent technological developments in electronics and computer made sEMG emerged as a subject of extensive research particularly in kinesiology, rehabilitation, and occupational and sports medicine. Most of the applications of sEMG are based on its use as a measure of activation time of muscle, a way of measuring muscle contraction profile, a measure of muscle contraction power, or as a measure of muscle mass fatigue (Hong, 2012). Just a few research articles applying sEMG techniques were released in the early 1950s. Today, over 2500 research publications appear each year.

The expansion of sEMG literature and the availability of appropriate instrumentation and techniques might suggest that understanding of the procedures utilised in recording the sEMG transmission and the relevant analysis strategies must be complete. However, the meaning of the signal remains questionable, and there are few sources accessible to help the novice Electromyographer be familiar with physiological and biophysical foundation sEMG, characteristics of the arrangement, signal analysis techniques, and appropriate sEMG applications (Alf Nachemson, 1983).

Sports technology studies on exercise equipment frequently use sEMG. Studies that use sEMG in sciences of the sport are mainly related to the determination of the system of contraction and relaxation of muscles as well as dealing with the evolution of accidental injuries. The data obtained from these studies can be used in the following areas: evaluation of the technical development, the establishment of the suitable exercise programmes follow up for the progress of the sportsmen in picking out skills (Hayden et al., 2005).

## 2.18 Skin Preparation in sEMG Studies

Preparation of the skin is essential to prevent skin impairment and receive a suitable signal. Before placing the electrodes on the skin, it must be guaranteed that the skin is clean and dry. The skin must be washed using gel, cream or perhaps alcohol and should be dried out (Zipp, 1982; Steele et al., 2012). If necessary, excess hair should be shaved. Cleansing the skin is advantageous to provide sEMG recordings with low noise levels. Appropriate planning of the skin assures removing body hair, oils and flaky skin layers and, as a result, reduces the impedance of the electrode-gel-skin interface. Shaving, wetting and rubbing with alcoholic beverages, acetone or ether are in many cases considered in cleaning the skin (Merletti et al., 2001).

Proper skin preparation and electrode positioning are essential components in acquiring high-quality sEMG measurements. Two key strategies control electrode preparations: 1) electrode contact must be stable; 2) skin impedance must be reduced. While there are no general guidelines for skin preparations, the kind of application and the required top quality signal usually determine the extent of the skin preparations (Fauth et al., 2010). For example, provided a targeted test movement is relatively static or unstable and only qualitative reading is desired, a simple alcohol cleaning around the area of attention is sufficient (Fauth et al., 2010). However, if the dynamic conditions present risk of the introduction of movement skin impairment like in walking, running or other planned accelerated changes, a thorough preparation is required. Some sEMG systems have an impedance checking circuit that sends an imperceptible burst of current through the electrodes, and controlled measurements are correlated to a known impedance level to indicate the quality of the electrode contacts (Fauth et al., 2010).

## 2.19 Electrode Material, Size, Montage and Positioning in EMG Studies

Surface electrodes are usually made of silver/silver chloride (Ag/AgCl), silver chloride (AgCl), silver (Ag) or perhaps gold (Au). Electrodes made from Ag/AgCl are often preferred to the others, as they are almost non-polarizable electrodes, which means that the electrode-skin impedance is a level of resistance and not a capacitance (Merletti et al., 2001). Therefore, the surface electrodes are probably less sensitive to comparative movements between the electrode surface area and the skin. Additionally, these types of electrodes provide a highly steady interface with the skin once electrolyte solution (for case in point gel) is interposed between the skin and the electrode (Merletti et al., 2001). Such a stable electrode-skin interface ensures high transmission to noise ratios.

The electrode should be placed on a motor point and the tendon insertion or two motor points along the longitudinal midline of the muscle. The longitudinal axis of the electrode should be lined up parallel to the length of the muscle tissue fibres. When an electrode is positioned on the skin, the recognition surface comes in contact with the electrolytes in the skin (Aparicio, 2005). In localising the site of recognition of the electrode on the epidermis, a variety of approaches have been used: 1) over the motor stage; 2) equidistant from the engine point; 3) near the electric motor point; 4) on the mid-point of the muscle belly; 5) on the visual part of the muscle mass belly; 6) at regular distances of osteological research points; and 7) without precision with respect to the placement at all (Hendrix et al., 2009).

In conclusion, sEMG is a helpful way in the analysis of muscle mass activity. However, its effectiveness is related to correct electrode placement, adequate skin preparation, and suitable recording instrumentation. Also, it is mandatory to recognise identify skin problems which may alter sEMG indicators and choose a particular blocking procedure before any additional evaluation (Geddes, 1972).

# CHAPTER 3

# METHODOLOGY

## 3.1 Design of the Study

The present study employed experimental design –randomised controlled trial before and after interventional study in which the participants were categorised into two different intervention groups. The following figure explains the processes involved in conducting this study.

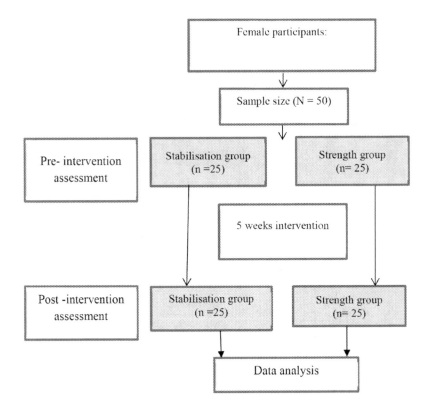

Figure 3.1: Research Framework

## 3.2 Study Population and Subject

For this study, 50 healthy female participants whose ages range from 19 to 24 years were chosen. The participants were students recruited from the

Faculty of Health Sciences, Universiti Sutan Zainal Abidin. These students volunteered to participate in this study. Participants with normal Body Mass Index (BMI) between 18.5 and 24.9 kg/m$^2$ who are in good health with no current or previous low back problems (James et al., 2002) were included in the study. Any participant with current low back or lower extremity pain or any recent surgery was excluded.

## 3.3 Study Sites

All interventions and questionnaire filling were carried out at the Physiotherapy Unit, Faculty of Health Science, Universiti Sultan Zainal Abidin.

## 3.4 Sample Size Calculation

The sample size was calculated using UCSF online Sample Size Calculator available at http://www.sample-size.net/sample-size-study-paired-t-test/. Comparison of the mean of EMG on rectus abdominis, gluteus medius and external oblique of dependent sample was applied based on the available and most comparable previous studies (Ekstrom et al. 2007; Ekstrom et al. 2008; Distefano et al. 2009; Okubo et al. 2010; Oliver et al. 2010; Selkowitz et al. 2013) (see Table 3.1).

The sample size calculation on EMG findings of one arm;

i. For rectus abdominis, n=21 participants based on

    alpha = 0.05

    power = 0.8

    standard deviation = 13

estimated mean difference = 8

ii. For the external oblique, the sample size is 21, based on

alpha = 0.05

power = 0.8

standard deviation = 26

estimated mean difference = 16

iii. For the gluteus medius, the sample is 24 participants in one arm only, based on

alpha = 0.05

power = 0.8

standard deviation = 42

estimated mean difference = 24

Table 3.1: Mean and standard deviation from previous studies

| Name of muscle | Mean and SD | Reference |
|---|---|---|
| Rectus Abdominis | (43.8+-14.3) (34+-13) | Ekstrom et al. (2007); Okubo et al. (2010). |
| External Oblique | (87.0+-36.1) (69+-26) | Ekstrom et al. (2007); Okubo et al. (2010). |
| Gluteus Medius | (43.5+-14.7) (81+-42) | Destifan et al. (2009); Selkowitz et al. (2013). |

## 3.5 Equipment

The following were the sEMG and other relevant equipment used in measuring the muscle activities in this study.

1. Bicycle (to warm up)

2. Razor (for shaving of hair which was performed if necessary)

3. Measuring tape (to put the electrodes in the exact area)

4. 70% isopropyl alcohol (to clean the site of electrode placement

5. Dual disposable silver/silver chloride surface recording electrodes (to record EMG)

6. Bioelectrical device (to measure weight and body fat)

7. 3V battery (for bioelectrical power supply)

8. Checklist form (to record the participant's background and data)

9. Myo Trac Infinity

## 3.6 Procedures and Exercises

The procedures employed in the present study are explained as follows.

1. Before electrode placement, each participant was acquainted with the procedures by being instructed and by practising the muscle tests and exercises performed. The researcher taught all the participants on how to perform each exercise using explanations and pictures.

2. Participants were trained on wearing suitable clothes.

3. Participants were warmed-up using bicycles before starting the exercise programme.

4. The sites of electrode placements were prepared by abrading the skin with fine sandpaper and cleansing the area with 70% isopropyl alcohol. Hair shaving was also performed when necessary.

5. Dual disposable silver/silver chloride surface recording electrodes were applied.

6. EMG data were collected from the rectus abdominis, external oblique, lumbar multifidus, gluteus maximus and gluteus medius.

Table 3.2: **Exercises Modalities under Strengthening Training Programme**

| Name of exercise | Muscle | How to perform | Reference |
|---|---|---|---|
| Full Crunches | Rectus Abdominis | Lie on your back on an exercise mat or bed. Bend both knees until your feet are flat on the floor. With your feet away from the floor, raise your upper body and shoulders to around 30 degrees off the floor. Rise and stop when your elbows reach your thighs. The entire curl up should take approximately 30s. | Koumantakis et al. (2005); Monfort-Escamilla et al. (2006); Teyhen et al. (2008); Hussain & Sharma (2008); Youdas et al. (2008); Pañego et al. (2009); Contreras & Schoenfeld (2011). |

| | | | |
|---|---|---|---|
| Side Crunches | External Oblique | Start out by lying on your back on the floor and turn both of your knees to the right. Slowly lift your shoulders off the floor and move your body straight up and then back down to the floor as if you were doing a regular crunch. Make sure that you keep your knees turned to the right as you do the crunch. | Koumantakis et al. (2005); Escamilla et al. (2006); Hussain & Sharma (2008); Monfort Pañego et al. (2009); Contreras & Schoenfeld (2011). |
| Lumbar Full Extension | Multifidus | Lie on your stomach and put your arms in front of your chest. Take your body up to a fully extended position. Your legs should be fully extended. | Arokoski et al. (2001); Stevens et al. (2007); Ekstrom et al. (2008); *Okubo et al. (2010).* |
| Hip Extension | Gluteus Maximus | Lie down; you can put your forehead on your hand or put a towel underneath your forehead. Lift your thigh off the ground and extend the leg. | *Selkowitz et al. (2013); Moon et al. (2013).* |
| Hip Abduction | Gluteus Medius | Lie on your side on an exercise mat or bed in a starting position. With knees fully extended, slowly abduct while keeping the knees extended. Stop at 30% of hip abduction and return slowly. | Serner et al. (2013). |

## Table 3.3: **Exercises Modalities under Stabilisation Training Programme**

| Name of exercise | Muscle | How to perform | Reference |
|---|---|---|---|
| Curl up | Rectus Abdominis | You need to lie on your back on an exercise mat or bed. Bend both knees until your feet are flat on the floor. With your feet away from the floor, lift your head and shoulders until your shoulder blades are off the floor. Hold for a moment at the top of the movement, and then slowly lower your back and hold on 5s. | Sarti et al. (1996); Koumantakis et al. (2005); Escamilla et al. (2006); Youdas et al. (2008); Teyhen et al. (2008); Monfort-Pañego et al. (2009); *Okubo et al. (2010).* |
| Plank Side | External Oblique | Lie on your side and brace your core muscles. Raise yourself up on the side of one foot and with your elbows raise your trunk off the floor and hold on 5s. | Koumantakis et al. (2005); Escamilla et al. (2006); Ekstrom et al. (2007); Teyhen et al. (2008); Ekstrom, et al. (2008); Youdas et al. (2008); Monfort-Pañego et al. (2009); *Okubo et al. (2010)*; Luque-Suárez et al. (2012); Garcia et al. (2013). |
| Back Bridge | Multifidus | Lie on your back with your knees bent, placing your heels close to your buttocks. Keep your arms at your sides with palms down, squeeze your gluteus and raise your hips off the floor to get into the bridge position and hold on 5s. | *Callaghan et al. (1998); Kendall et al. (2005)*; Koumantakis et al. (2005); Stevens et al. (2007); Ekstrom et al. (2008); Luque-Suárez et al. (2012). |

| Plank hip extension | Gluteus Maximus | Start by lying prone on your elbows in planks with trunk, hips, and knees in neutral alignment (left). Lift your dominant leg off the ground, flex the knee of your dominant leg and extend the hip past the neutral hip alignment by bringing the heel in. | *Distefano et al. (2009); Selkowitz et al. (2013).* |
|---|---|---|---|
| Plank hip Abduction | Gluteus Medius | Dominant leg down. Begin with a side plank position. You are reminded to keep shoulders, hips, knees, and ankles in line bilaterally, and then rise to plank position with your hips lifted off the ground to achieve a neutral alignment with your trunk, hips, and knees. While balancing on your elbows and feet, raise the top leg into abduction (right) for one beat and then lower your leg for one beat. | Serner et al. (2013). |

## NOTES:

i.    Each exercise modality consists of three cycles, and each cycle should be performed 8 times approximately within 1 minute.

ii.   Rest periods of 10 seconds were allowed between cycles of the exercises and 1 minute between specific exercise modalities.

iii.  An overall one hour was needed for each type of exercise modality to complete the task for one participant.

iv. One participant performed and assessed in the morning and one in the afternoon.

The exercises were performed by participants three times a week for a period of 5 weeks consecutively (Ingersoll & Knight, 1991; Stone & Coulter 1994; Cordova et al., 1995; Ekstrom et al., 2007; Ekstrom et al., 2008).

## 3.7 EMG measurement

For the rectus abdominis muscle, the electrodes were placed 3 cm lateral and 3 cm superior to the umbilicus (Criswell, 2010). The electrodes were placed midway between the anterior superior iliac spine and the rib cage for the external oblique and abdominis muscle (Danneels et al. 2002; Criswell 2010).

For the lumbar multifidus muscle, the electrodes were placed 2 cm lateral to the lumbosacral junction (Danneels et al. 2002). The electrodes for the gluteus medius muscle were placed anterosuperior to the gluteus maximus muscle and just inferior to the iliac crest on the lateral side of the pelvis (Criswell, 2010).

For the gluteus maximus muscle, electrodes were placed in the centre of the muscle belly between the lateral edge of the sacrum and the superior poster edge of the greater trochanter (Criswell, 2010). A reference electrode was placed over the anterior superior iliac spine (Ekstrom et al., 2007).

## 3.8 Statistical Analysis

The data entry and analysis were performed using XLSTAT 2014 add-in software, USA. The independent t-test, also defined as the two-sample t-test, independent samples t-test or student's t-test, is an inferential mathematical test that measures whether there is a statistically significant difference between the means of two separate groups. The null hypothesis for the independent t-test states that the population means obtained from the two separate groups are equal as suggested by Heeren and D'Agostino (1987).

The independent t-test was applied to compare the efficacy of the post-measurement of the muscle activations between the strengthening and the stabilisation exercise programmes on all the measured muscles in the study. The paired t-test analysis was also employed earlier in this study to determine whether there is a significant difference between the pre- and post-training exercise modalities. The level of significance was set at 0.05.

## 4.1 Introduction

This chapter describes the results and interprets the data based on the objectives of the study. The results and analysis are provided in consecutive order. The initial results are the baseline characteristics of the participants and its comparison between the two intervention groups (see Table 4.1). The results revealed that both groups were not significantly different regarding their age, weight, height and BMI. This indicates that their characteristics at baseline were almost similar and comparable.

Later, the results and the discussions on the effect of strengthening training on the five muscles examined in this study are projected, followed by the results and the explanations of the effect of stabilisation training on the aforementioned muscles. Finally, the comparative efficacy of the muscle activities of the two training programmes in females (strengthening and stabilisation) is presented and discussed.

Table 4.1: The baseline characteristics of the female participants

| Baseline characteristics | Strengthening (n=25) Mean | Stabilisation (n=25) Mean | Mean difference | t statistic | p-value [a] |
|---|---|---|---|---|---|
| Age (years) | 18.8 | 18.8 | 0.7 | 0.5 | 0.096 |
| Height (cm) | 155.54 | 158.18 | 7.7 | 1.69 | 0.205 |
| Weight (kg) | 48.44 | 49.79 | 8.1 | 1.04 | 0.091 |
| Body Mass Index (kg/m$^2$) | 19.9 | 20.04 | 2.49 | 0.47 | 0.075 |

[a]Independent t-test

## 4.2 The Effect of Strengthening Training Programme on the Muscle Activities in Females

### 4.2.1 Results

Table 4.2 presents the descriptive statistics of the pre-and post-strengthening training programme (STTP) on the evaluated muscles. The intervention period (pre-and post), the number of participants, the minimum, maximum, and mean scores, as well as the standard deviation of each variable, are shown. It can be observed from the table that the means of the post-intervention measurement were greater than the pre-measurement, indicating that the means of muscle activations of the post-measurement were considerably higher compared to the pre-measurement.

Table 4.2: Descriptive Statistics of Pre-and Post-Strengthening Training Intervention Programme (STTP) on the Muscles (n=25)

| Muscle types | Intervention Period | n | Minimum | Maximum | Mean | SD |
|---|---|---|---|---|---|---|
| **Trunk muscles** | | | | | | |
| Rectus Abdominis | Pre | 25 | 19.76 | 128.55 | 80.31 | 24.26 |
| | Post | 25 | 94.01 | 169.47 | 142.53 | 18.08 |
| External Oblique | Pre | 25 | 35.14 | 119.30 | 76.51 | 23.94 |
| | Post | 25 | 93.31 | 178.56 | 141.79 | 24.99 |
| Multifidus | Pre | 25 | 53.48 | 122.26 | 83.79 | 17.37 |
| | Post | 25 | 92.45 | 154.96 | 133.73 | 22.39 |
| **Hip muscles** | | | | | | |
| Gluteus Maximus | Pre | 25 | 12.32 | 130.58 | 83.61 | 21.07 |
| | Post | 25 | 99.05 | 174.78 | 134.74 | 23.29 |
| Gluteus Medius | Pre | 25 | 18.34 | 126.32 | 83.12 | 23.00 |
| | Post | 25 | 86.29 | 169.34 | 145.86 | 19.95 |

SD=standard deviation

Table 4.3 reveals the inferential statistics results. It can be seen that there was the statistically significant difference between the pre-and post-strengthening training on the muscle activations in all the evaluated muscles of rectus abdominis, external oblique, multifidus, gluteus maximus, and gluteus medius ($p<0.001$). This result suggests that STTP intervention was effective in improving the selected muscles activations of the participants examined in the study.

Table 4.3: Inferential Statistics of the Pre-and Post-Test of the Strengthening Training Intervention Programme (STTP) on the Muscles (n=25)

| Muscle types | t(obs.) | t(crtcl) | DF | D statistic | p value[a] |
|---|---|---|---|---|---|
| **Trunk muscles** | | | | | |
| Rectus Abdominis | -10.28 | 2.01 | 48 | -62.22 | 0.001 |
| External Oblique | -9.433 | 2.01 | 48 | -65.28 | 0.001 |
| Multifidus | -8.81 | 2.01 | 48 | -49.94 | 0.001 |
| **Hip muscles** | | | | | |
| Gluteus Maximus | -8.14 | 2.01 | 48 | -51.13 | 0.001 |
| Gluteus Medius | -10.3 | 2.01 | 48 | -62.74 | 0.001 |

DF = degree of freedom, [a]Paired t-test

## 4.2.2 Discussion

The results of the STTP intervention and the EMG activities of the muscle examined in the present study indicate that the STTP was effective in improving the selected muscles of the participants. The evidence provided in Table 4.2 and Table 4.3 suggests that trunk and hip muscles of the female participants in the study have responded to the implemented training programme. The results further indicate that STTP could be useful as rehabilitation exercises in female participants.

Kankaanpää, Taimela, Laaksonen, Hänninen, and Airaksinen (1998) examined the value of specific trunk, hip, muscle strengthening, and backing training in the prevention of injuries. It was concluded from their findings that strengthening training is vital in reducing the prevalence of injury and occurrence of LBP. It has also been reported that weakness and poor stamina from the lumbar and gluteus muscle tissue in people with lower extremity accidental injuries and LBP could be effectively improved through STTP interventions (Biering-sØrensen, 1984; Leetun, Ireland, Willson, Ballantyne, & Davis, 2004).

Muscle strength is a wide term that encompasses the capacity of the contractile tissue to generate force and resultant tension with regards to the demands placed on the muscle. Strengthening training is described as a systematic strategy of a tissue or muscle group lifting, lowering or controlling heavy loads (resistance) for a comparatively low amount of repetitions or over a short time span (Sozen, 2010).

Researchers have indicated that the deep fibers of multifidus and transverse abdominis are among the initial muscles required to become active when there is a postural change from rapid extremity movements (Hodges, 1999). The rectus abdominis, external oblique, and internal oblique muscles are large, multi-segmental global muscles and are vital catalysts for supporting the spine against postural perturbations. The transverse abdominis is the deepest of the abdominal muscles and responds exclusively to postural perturbations.

It has been established that activation and function of these muscles could substantially be improved through the STTP interventions in patients with LBP (Hodges, 1999). Some authors have similarly documented that STTP is useful in the improvement of postural control and stability for a long-term benefit (Hides, Jull, & Richardson, 2001).

Muscular strength is perceived to be the ability of a muscle or group of muscles to produce force and hence muscular strength is enhanced with STTP. STTP is applied in physical fitness and the prevention and restoration of musculoskeletal impairments (Van Tulder, Malmivaara, Esmail, & Koes, 1999). For example, low back extensor muscle strength is a significant determinant of low back health, and thus STTP serve as a means of rehabilitation of the lower back, avoidance of injury, and as a constituent of physical fitness exercise programmes to improve performance standards (Callaghan, Gunning, & McGill, 1998; Gracovetsky, 2010).

The findings of the current study have further indicated that STTP intervention is effective in increasing the muscles activations among healthy female participants. An increase in muscle activations is associated with the capacity of the muscles to respond effectively to the demands placed upon them. The back extensors serve as crucial muscles during raising and bending actions. Norris (2008) indicated that these muscles act both to stretch the spine and to stabilise the flexion motion created by the trunk when weight is being raised.

This explanation could be comprehended by many people with LBP possess weak low back muscles which hinder or restricts higher muscle activations (Graves et al., 1994). Hence, the current findings could be extended to help the LBP patients in enhancing the strength of their activities.

## 4.3 The Effect of Stabilisation Training Programme on Muscle Activitions in Females

### 4.3.1 Results

Table 4.4 reveals the descriptive statistics of the pre-and post SBTP on the evaluated muscles. The period of the intervention (pre-and post), the number of participants, the minimum, maximum, and mean scores, as well as the standard deviation of each variable, are displayed in Table 4.4. It can be noticed from the table that the average of the post-intervention measurement is larger than the pre-measurement, demonstrating that the average muscle activations of the post-measurement are considerably higher compared to the pre-measurement.

Table 4.4: Descriptive Statistics of the Pre-and Post
SBTP on the assessed muscles (n=25)

| Muscle types | Intervention period | n | Minimum | Maximum | Mean | SD |
|---|---|---|---|---|---|---|
| **Trunk muscles** | | | | | | |
| Rectus Abdominis | Pre | 25 | 27.84 | 438.96 | 132.13 | 134.42 |
| | Post | 25 | 78.76 | 1933.23 | 372.87 | 439.46 |
| External Oblique | Pre | 25 | 46.16 | 497.65 | 117.15 | 104.89 |
| | Post | 25 | 91.96 | 1378.43 | 322.24 | 358.39 |
| Multifidus | Pre | 25 | 30.88 | 377.86 | 110.84 | 97.73 |
| | Post | 25 | 56.72 | 1409.28 | 325.28 | 334.10 |
| **Hip muscles** | | | | | | |
| Gluteus Maximus | Pre | 25 | 21.12 | 501.94 | 136.29 | 146.31 |
| | Post | 25 | 76.02 | 1259.33 | 342.20 | 292.61 |
| Gluteus Medius | Pre | 25 | 15.07 | 494.68 | 142.46 | 144.57 |
| | Post | 25 | 88.21 | 1031.67 | 313.50 | 197.58 |

SD=standard deviation

Table 4.5 shows the inferential statistics of the comparison carried out as a follow-up for the *t*-test. In the table, t observed, t critical, the degree of freedom, and the difference between the pre-and post-evaluations, as well as the significant levels, are indicated.

It can be observed that there was a statistically significant difference between the pre-and post-evaluations on the muscle activations in all the assessed muscles of rectus abdominis, external oblique, multifidus, gluteus maximus, and gluteus medius ($p < 0.05$). This result implies that SBTP intervention was also efficient in increasing the aforementioned muscles activations of the female participants observed in the study.

Table 4.5: Pre-and Post-test Inferential Statistics of
the SBTP on the Evaluated Muscles (n=25)

| Muscle types | t(obs.) | t(crtcl) | DF | D statistic | p value[a] |
|---|---|---|---|---|---|
| **Trunk muscles** | | | | | |
| Rectus Abdominis | -2.62 | 2.01 | 48 | -240.7 | 0.011 |
| External Oblique | -2.75 | 2.01 | 48 | -205.1 | 0.008 |
| Multifidus | -3.08 | 2.01 | 48 | -214.4 | 0.003 |
| **Hip muscles** | | | | | |
| Gluteus Maximus | -3.15 | 2.01 | 48 | -205.9 | 0.002 |
| Gluteus Medius | -3.49 | 2.01 | 48 | -171 | 0.001 |

DF = degree of freedom, [a]Paired t-test

## 4.3.2 Discussion

The overall findings of the SBTP intervention and the EMG activities of the muscle experiment in the present study demonstrated that the SBTP is efficient in the enhancement of muscle activations. The proof given in Table 4.4 and Table 4.5 showed that trunk and hip muscles of the female participants in the study have improved after implementation of the programme. The results indicated that SBTP could also be effective as rehabilitation exercises in female participants.

The purposes of stabilisation exercise are to develop muscular motor sequences to enhance spinal balance, prevent irregular micro-motion, and decrease related pain. Different investigations focusing on muscle onset and EMG sequences have proposed that some specific muscles are an essential to measure of stability (Richardson, Jull, Hodges, & Hides, 1999). Some studies documented that all muscles perform a role in providing spine stability and that the motor sequences of co-contraction between the entire supplement of muscles are of absolute significance to secure stability and reduce pain (Gardner-Morse, Stokes, and Laible, 1995; Cholewicki, and McGill, 1996). Despite the fact that the exercises considered in this research are reported in the literature as targeting a distinct muscle group, EMG studies demonstrated that the exercises could stimulate combinations of muscles in a manner that reinforces overall spinal stability (Hides, Jull, & Richardson, 2001).

Some investigations indicated that training programmes could be devised to stimulate the spine muscles in a form that turns out to be efficient for some patients with LBP (Hides, Richardson, & Jull, 1996; O'sullivan, Phyty, Twomey, & Allison, 1997). Similarly, Delitto, Erhard, and Bowling, (1995) and Ogon et al. (1997) indicated that the observation of abnormal movement patterns during active trunk motion is important in the analysis of lumbar Segmental Instability (LSI). The existence of abnormal movements may serve as incapacity to satisfactorily regulate lumbar movement and point to the need for stabilisation training. Patients with LSI have been referred to as a special subgroup of patients with LBP (Panjabi, Lydon, Vasavada, Grab, Crisco, & Dvorak, 1994; Delitto, Erhard, & Bowling, 1995). LSI has been interpreted as a situation in which there is a decline of rigidity between spinal movement portions, such that the commonly permitted external loads result in discomfort, impairment or otherwise renders neurologic structures at risk.

Training programmes devised to enhance spinal stabilisation have got acceptance in the conventional rehabilitation of patients with LBP. However, evidence for the efficacy of this technique is inadequate and ambiguous (BenDebba, Torgerson, & Long, 2000). The few investigations that have considered specific stabilisation exercise programmes among patients with LBP in more homogenous populations have demonstrated some promising effects. O'sullivan, Phyty, Twomey, & Allison, (1997) randomised patients with chronic and recurrent LBP who had a radiologic diagnosis of spondylolysis or spondylolisthesis to obtain either stabilisation exercises or usual care given by a practitioner. The authors have discovered statistically significant reductions in pain at a 30-month follow-up.

In another development, Hides, Richardson, & Jull (1996) examined participants with acute, early-rate occurrence of unilateral LBP, comparing stabilisation exercises specifically aiming at multifidus muscle with regular medical care. No substantial deviations in impairment or discomfort were detected after four weeks, but the stabilisation group felt relatively fewer recurrences at a 2 to 3-year follow-up. These researchers illustrated that a particular stabilisation exercise programme might be useful for specific subgroups of patients. These investigations are in agreement with the findings of the present study that SBTP is efficient in enhancing the muscle activities among healthy female participants which could likewise be alluded in the rehabilitation of LBP patients.

## 4.4 The Comparative Efficacy of Stabilisation and Strengthening Training Intervention Programme on the Muscle Activities of Post Intervention in Females

### 4.4.1 Results

Table 4.6 presents the descriptive statistics of the relative effectiveness of SBTP and STTP intervention programme in the improvement of muscles at the post evaluation. The type of training programme (strengthening and stabilisation), the total number of participants, the minimum, maximum, mean and scores, as well as the standard deviation of each variable are illustrated. It can be noticed from the table that the means of the post-intervention measurement of the SBTP was larger than the STTP across all the post measurements, indicating that the muscle activations of the stabilisation modalities remained substantially higher as opposed to the STTP after the interventions in females.

Table 4.6: Descriptive statistics of the comparative efficacy of stabilisation and strengthening training intervention programme on the muscles

| Muscles types | Training Programmes | n | Minimum | Maximum | Mean | SD |
|---|---|---|---|---|---|---|
| **Trunk muscles** | | | | | | |
| Rectus Abdominis | Strengthening | 25 | 94.01 | 169.47 | 142.53 | 18.08 |
| | Stabilisation | 25 | 78.76 | 1933.23 | 372.87 | 439.46 |
| External Oblique | Strengthening | 25 | 93.31 | 178.56 | 141.79 | 24.99 |
| | Stabilisation | 25 | 91.96 | 1378.43 | 322.24 | 358.39 |
| Multifidus | Strengthening | 25 | 92.45 | 154.96 | 133.73 | 22.39 |
| | Stabilisation | 25 | 56.72 | 1409.28 | 325.28 | 334.10 |
| **Hip muscles** | | 25 | | | | |
| Gluteus Maximus | Strengthening | 25 | 99.05 | 174.78 | 134.74 | 23.29 |
| | Stabilisation | 25 | 76.02 | 1259.33 | 342.20 | 292.61 |
| Gluteus Medius | Strengthening | 25 | 86.29 | 169.34 | 145.86 | 19.95 |
| | Stabilisation | 25 | 88.21 | 1031.67 | 313.50 | 197.58 |

SD=standard deviation

Table 4.7 displays the inferential statistics of comparison between STBP and STTP. From the table, t observed, t critical, the degree of freedom, the difference between the SBTP and STTP at the post evaluations, and the significant levels are demonstrated. It can be seen that there was a statistically significant difference between the SBTP and STTP on the muscle activations in all the evaluated muscles of rectus abdominis, external oblique, multifidus, gluteus maximus, and gluteus medius ($p < 0.05$). This finding signifies that SBTP intervention was more effective compared to STTP in improving the muscles activations of female participants evaluated in the study.

Table 4.7: Inferential statistics for the comparative efficacy of stabilisation and strengthening training intervention programme on the muscles assessed

| Muscle types | t(obs.) | t(crtcl) | DF | D statistic | p value[a] |
|---|---|---|---|---|---|
| **Trunk muscles** | | | | | |
| Rectus Abdominis | -2.62 | 2.01 | 48 | -230.3 | 0.011 |
| External Oblique | -2.51 | 2.01 | 48 | -180.5 | 0.015 |
| Multifidus | -2.86 | 2.01 | 48 | -191.6 | 0.006 |
| **Hip muscles** | | | | | |
| Gluteus Maximus | -3.53 | 2.01 | 48 | -207.5 | 0.009 |
| Gluteus Medius | -4.22 | 2.01 | 48 | -167.6 | 0.001 |

DF = degree of freedom, [a]Independent t-test

Figure 4.1 to Figure 4.5 highlight the comparable effectiveness pattern analysis between SBTP and STTP in the improvement of all the muscles assessed in the study during post-intervention assessment. From the figures, it can be noted that the SBTP intervention recorded higher muscles activations across all the muscles of the rectus abdominis, external oblique, multifidus, gluteus maximus, and gluteus medius. The greater rate of activations observed in SBTP interventions can be attributed to the effectiveness of the training programme in targeting the evaluated muscles. The result shows that the SBTP intervention was better in stimulating all the muscles evaluated compared with the STTP.

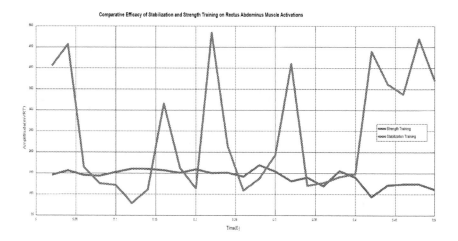

Figure 4.1: Descriptive analysis of comparative efficacy between SBTP and
STTP in the improvement of Rectus Abdominis muscle activation

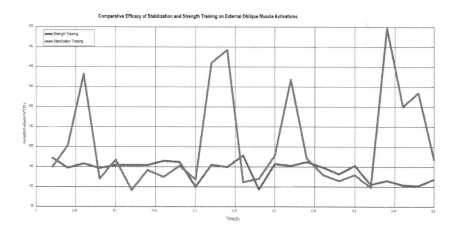

Figure 4.2: Descriptive analysis of comparative effectiveness between SBTP
and STTP in the development of External Oblique muscle activation

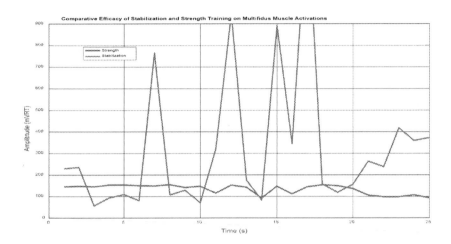

Figure 4.3: Descriptive analysis of comparative efficacy between SBTP and STTP in the improvement of Multifidus muscle activation

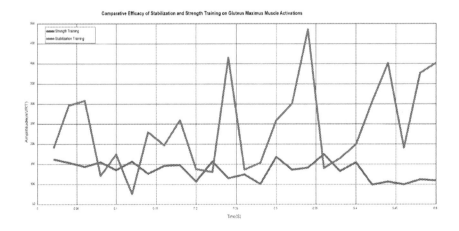

Figure 4.4: Descriptive analysis of comparative efficacy between SBTP and STTP in the improvement of Gluteus Maximus muscle activation

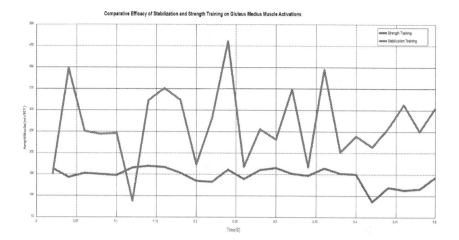

Figure 4.5: Descriptive analysis of comparative efficacy between SBTP and STTP in the improvement of Gluteus Medius muscle activation

## 4.4.2 Discussion

The overall results of the comparative effectiveness of SBTP and STTP intervention programmes in improving muscles at the post-session of the EMG activities of the muscle experiments in the study have indicated that the SBTP was more effective in the improvement of the participants' muscles when compared with the STTP. The evidence presented in Table 4.6, Table 4.7 and Figures 4.1 to Figure 4.5 showed that trunk and hip muscles of the female participants in the study have improved more in the SBTP intervention than in the STTP. The results suggest that SBTP could be highly useful as rehabilitation exercises of related LBP in females.

The findings of the current study are in line with some of the previous studies which reported that specific stabilisation exercises could be advantageous in LBP patients (May, & Johnson, 2008). Byström, Rasmussen-Barr, and Grooten (2013) concluded that SBTP is beneficial in the long-term period in alleviating disability with regards to pain at a moderate level.

Some studies have also suggested that exercise modalities can be designed to improve the supporting muscles of the spine in a valuable pattern for some patients with LBP (Hides, Richardson, & Jull, 1996; O'sullivan, Phyty, Twomey, & Allison, 1997).

Other studies pointed out that the study of irregular movement patterns during active trunk motion is crucial in the examination of LSI (Likewise, Delitto, Erhard, & Bowling, 1995; Ogon et al, 1997). It has been stated that the general aims of stabilisation exercise are to increase muscular motor orders to improve spinal support, counter abnormal micro-motion and decrease associated pain (Gardner-Morse, Stokes, & Laible, 1995). Therefore, it is expected that some researchers who studied muscle origin and EMG sequences recommended that lumbar muscles are better stimulated through the application of some stability exercises (Richardson, Jull, Hodges, & Hides, 1999).

Ferreira et al. (2007) studied three sorts of rehabilitation programmes consisting of regular exercises, stabilisation exercises, and manual therapy about pain and functional impairment in patients with CLBP. The results revealed that regular exercises in the short-time period lead to more pain than relief in the corresponding methods, while stabilisation training projects a long-term decline in pain and disability compared with all other methods. Similarly, Cairns, Foster, and Wright (2006) conducted a study to examine the physical stability and physical therapy training in women with LBP. It was concluded from their findings that both training modalities are effective in reducing pain intensity among the groups.

The results of the present study revealed that the participants in the SBTP group experienced a better improved lumbar muscle activation determined by spectral EMG, which could as well have had an impact in increasing the overall endurance of the muscles and consequently have an effect on reducing back pain severity. In the same vein, a study established that for individuals who have a record of back pain connected with abdominal and spine muscle weakness, their selection of training programme must be tailored towards stabilising these groups of muscles to minimise the present and subsequent pain (Mamashli, Mahdavinejad, & Goodarzi, 2014).

Therefore, the present results show that improved lumbar activations could be associated with better outcome of the observed higher muscles activation. The improvement in lumbar muscle activations capacity in the SBTP intervention group is in conformity with the results of earlier studies (Mayer, Kondraske, Mooney, Carmichael, & Butsch, 1989; Roy, De Luca, Emley, & Buijs, 1995; Mooney, Gulick, Perlman, Levy, Pozos, Leggett, & Resnick, 1997)

## 4.5 Limitation of the Study

This study has not been conducted on a large-scale due to time, logistic and financial limitations. The study also has faced several technical limitations ranging from managing the subjects, provision of suitable laboratory equipment, to congestion in the laboratory due to high demand by other students.

The psychological condition of the subjects is another limitation in this study because the researcher had to ensure that every subject is in a good mood to allow smooth recording without unnecessary errors. It took the researcher about three months to provide the electrodes that were used for recording data in the laboratory.

# CHAPTER 5

## SUMMARY AND CONCLUSION

## Introduction

This chapter comprises summary and conclusion of the overall findings of the study. The chapter also presents some practical implications and recommendations for physiotherapists, trainers and other stakeholders involved in the clinical spectrum. Suggestions for further study have also been provided.

## 5.1 Summary

The present study, after a rigorous and careful review of various literatures in clinical, physiotherapist perspective and some other related sports and exercise dimensions, discovered that there is a relatively limited number of studies that attempted to study and compare between strengthening and stabilisation training and other modalities among healthy participants to serve as an effective mechanism for reducing LBP in female patients. The study aims at drawing the attention of the physiotherapists, trainers and other stakeholders to determine the most appropriate training programme capable of giving maximum effects in developing and stimulating the lumbar muscles of female participants. This will consequently serve as a guide for the application of exercise programmes in the reduction and rehabilitations of LBP amongst female patients. To this effect, the study examined two main training programmes: STTP) and SBTP interventions. The effectiveness of these programmes in improving the targeted muscles activations has been considered in this study.

The objectives of this study were to critically examine the effectiveness of each training programme in improving the muscles activities of rectus abdominis, external oblique, multifidus, gluteus maximus and gluteus medius from pre and post evaluations and finally highlight the most effective training programme between the STTP and SBTP in the overall improvement of the activations of the aforementioned muscles.

The study adopted an experimental randomised control trial design and allotted the participants randomly into two different intervention groups: STTP and SBTP. A total of 50 healthy female participants with normal BMI and without any record of current or previous lower extremity or back problems with ages ranging from 19 to 24 years were recruited to participate in the study. The participants were divided into either STTP or SBTP and each group consisted of 25 participants. Both the STTP and SBTP groups performed a different set of exercises related to their peculiar training programme separately, and the initial measurement of the muscles activations was taken (pre-measurement). EMG data were collected from the five muscles (rectus abdominis, external oblique, multifidus, gluteus maximus, and gluteus medius). The readings from the EMG were compared after the five weeks interventions (post-measurement). A paired t-test and an independent t-test were applied to the data gathered to examine the differences between pre and post-measurement of both the STTP and the SBTP and compare the overall effect of the training programmes (post STTP and the post-readings of SBTP) on the targeted muscles respectively.

The overall findings of the STTP intervention and the EMG activities of the muscles examined in the present study have indicated that the STTP was effective in the improvement of the selected muscles of the participants. The STTP intervention results have suggested that the trunk and hip muscles of the female participants in the study have responded to the training programme implemented. Likewise, the results of the SBTP intervention and the EMG activities of the experimented muscles in the study have also demonstrated that the SBTP is efficient in improving the activations of the participants' muscles. The results further indicated that STTP and SBTP could be useful as rehabilitation exercises in female participants.

The overall results of the comparative effectiveness of SBTP and STTP intervention programme at the post EMG activities of the experimented muscles in the study have indicated that the SBTP was more effective in improving the activations of the participants' muscles when compared with the STTP. The study discovered that trunk and hip muscles of the female participants in the study have improved more in SBTP intervention than in STTP.

## 5.2 Conclusion

The results of the present study demonstrated that both the five-week strengthening and stabilisation training programmes implemented in the study are effective in improving the muscle activations of the female participants within the training intervention period. Nonetheless, the stabilisation intervention has appeared to be more effective in stimulating the selected muscles.

## 5.3 Practical Implication of the Study

The results suggested that SBTP could be more useful as rehabilitation exercises of related LBP in female participants than the STTP. Moreover, the study has shown that utilisation of sEMG signals in detecting muscles activations is helpful as it enables the researcher to accurately identify the best intervention training programme that can enhance the activations of the lumbar muscles amongst healthy female participants. This would, in the long run, apply to the female patients with a record of LBP. A CLBP patient's physical ailment can be restored after obtaining proper therapy, employing an appropriate and simple medical rehabilitation process. As a result, the patients' physical condition can revert to the earlier form.

From biomedical perspectives, physiological sensors are the principal elements of biosignal processing and electronic medical rehabilitation technique. The EMG biosensors denote the connection between biomedical signals and rehabilitations. Therefore, the application of this technology has enabled the identification of appropriate intervention programmes that could benefit physiotherapists in adopting the rehabilitation of female participants diagnosed with LBP.

# REFERENCES

Abenhaim, L., Rossignol, M., Valat, J. P., Nordin, M., Avouac, B., Blotman, F. & Vautravers, P. (2000). The role of activity in the therapeutic management of back pain: *Report of the International Paris Task Force on Back Pain. Spine, 25 (4) 312-335.*

Adams, M. A., Stefanakis, M., & Dolan, P. (2010). Healing of a painful intervertebral disc should not be confused with reversing disc degeneration: *implications for physical therapies for discogenic back pain. Clinical Biomechanics, 25(10), 961–971.*

Alaranta, H., Rytökoski, U., Rissanen, A., Talo, S., Rönnemaa, T., Puukka, P., ... Slätis, P. (1994). *Intensive Physical and Psychosocial Training Program for Patients with Chronic Low Back Pain; A Controlled Clinical Trial. Spine, 19(12), 1339–1349.*

Alkner, B. A., Tesch, P. A., & Berg, H. E. (2000). Quadriceps EMG/force relationship in knee extension and leg press. *Medicine and Science in Sports and Exercise, 32(2), 459–463.*

Anders, C., Scholle, H.-C., Wagner, H., Puta, C., Grassme, R., & Petrovitch, A. (2005). Trunk muscle co-ordination during gait: relationship between muscle function and acute low back pain. Pathophysiology, 12(4), 243–247.

Andersen, L. L., Andersen, C. H., Mortensen, O. S., Poulsen, O. M., Bjørnlund, I. B. T., & Zebis, M. K. (2010). Muscle activation and perceived loading during rehabilitation exercises: comparison of dumbbells and elastic resistance. Physical Therapy, 90(4), 538–549.

Andersson, G. B. J. (1999). Epidemiological features of chronic low-back pain. *The Lancet, 354(9178), 581–585.*

Andersson, G. B. J., Chaffin, D. B., & Pope, M. H. (1991). Occupational biomechanics of the lumbar spine. *Occupational Low Back Pain. St Louis, MO: Mosby, 20–43.*

Aparicio, M. A. V. (2005). *Electromiografía cinesiológica. Rehabilitación, 39(6), 255–264.*

Arab, A. M., & Ebrahimi, E. (2005). *Clinical trunk muscle endurance tests in subjects with and without low back pain. MJIRI.*

Arnau, J. M., Vallano, A., Lopez, A., Pellisé, F., Delgado, M. J., & Prat, N. (2006). A critical review of guidelines for low back pain treatment. *European Spine Journal, 15(5), 543–553.*

Arokoski, J. P. A., Kankaanpää, M., Valta, T., Juvonen, I., Partanen, J., Taimela, S., … Airaksinen, O. (1999). Back and hip extensor muscle function during therapeutic exercises. *Archives of Physical Medicine and Rehabilitation, 80(7), 842–850.*

Arokoski, J. P., Valta, T., Airaksinen, O., & Kankaanpää, M. (2001). Back and abdominal muscle function during stabilization exercises. *Archives of physical medicine and rehabilitation, 82 (8) 1089-1098.*

Arokoski, J. P., Valta, T., Kankaanpää, M., & Airaksinen, O. (2004). Activation of lumbar paraspinal and abdominal muscles during therapeutic exercises in chronic low back pain patients. *Archives of physical medicine and rehabilitation, 85(5), 823-832.*

Baars, H., Jöllenbeck, T., Humburg, H., & Schröder, J. (2007). Surface-electromyography: skin and subcutaneous fat tissue attenuate amplitude and frequency parameters. *In ISBS-Conference Proceedings Archive (Vol. 1).*

Balestra, G., Frassinelli, S., Knaflitz, M., & Molinari, F. (2001). Time-frequency analysis of surface myoelectric signals during athletic movement. *IEEE Engineering in Medicine and Biology Magazine, 20(6), 106–115.*

Baratta, R., Solomonow, M., Zhou, B. H., Letson, D., Chuinard, R., & D'ambrosia, R. (1988). Muscular coactivation: the role of the antagonist musculature in maintaining knee stability. *The American Journal of Sports Medicine, 16(2), 113–122.*

Barker, K. L., Shamley, D. R., & Jackson, D. (2004). Changes in the cross-sectional area of multifidus and psoas in patients with unilateral back pain: *the relationship to pain and disability. Spine, 29(22), E515–E519.*

Barrero, L. H., Hsu, Y.-H., Terwedow, H., Perry, M. J., Dennerlein, J. T., Brain, J. D., & Xu, X. (2006). *Prevalence and physical determinants of low back pain in a rural Chinese population. Spine, 31(23), 2728-2734.*

Basmajian, J. V, & De Luca, C. J. (1985). *Muscles alive: their functions revealed by electromyography. Williams & Wilkins.*

Beck, T. W., Housh, T., Fry, A. C., Cramer, J. T., Weir, J., Schilling, B., ... Moore, C. (2009). MMG-EMG cross spectrum and muscle fiber type. *International Journal of Sports Medicine, 30(7), 538–544.*

Beinart, N. A., Goodchild, C. E., Weinman, J. A., Ayis, S., & Godfrey, E. L. (2013). Individual and intervention-related factors associated with adherence to home exercise in chronic low back pain: a systematic review. *The Spine Journal, 13 (12) 1940-1950.*

Bekkering, G. E., Hendriks, H. J. M., Koes, B. W., Oostendorp, R. A. B., Ostelo, R., Thomassen, J. M. C., & Van Tulder, M. W. (2003). Dutch physiotherapy guidelines for low back pain. *Physiotherapy, 89(2), 82–96.*

Bell, D. G. (1993). The influence of air temperature on the EMG/force relationship of the quadriceps. *European Journal of Applied Physiology and Occupational Physiology, 67(3), 256–260.*

BenDebba, M., Torgerson, W. S., & Long, D. M. (2000). A validated, practical classification procedure for many persistent low back pain patients. *Pain, 87(1), 89-97.*

Bendix, A. F., Bendix, T., Haestrup, C., & Busch, E. (1998). A prospective, randomized 5-year follow-up study of functional restoration in chronic low back pain patients. *European Spine Journal, 7(2), 111–119.*

Bendix, T., Bendix, A., Labriola, M., Hæstrup, C., & Ebbehøj, N. (2000). Functional restoration versus outpatient physical training in chronic low back pain: a randomized comparative study. *Spine, 25(19), 2494-2500.*

Bergquist-Ullman, M., & Larsson, U. (1977). Acute low back pain in industry: a controlled prospective study with special reference to therapy and confounding factors. *Acta Orthopaedica Scandinavica, 48(sup170),* *1–117.*

Biering-sØrensen, F. (1984). Physical measurements as risk indicators for low-back trouble over a one-year period. *Spine, 9 (2) 106-119.*

Bigos, S., Bowyer, O., Braen, G., Brown, K., Deyo, R., Haldeman, S., ... Kido, D. (1994). Acute lower back problems in adults. Rockville, MD: *Agency for Health Care Policy and Research.*

Blumenstein, B., Bar-Eli, M., & Tenenbaum, G. (2002). *Brain and body in sport and exercise: Biofeedback applications in performance enhancement. John Wiley & Sons.*

Bogey, R., Cerny, K., & Mohammed, O. (2003). Repeatability of wire and surface electrodes in gait. *American Journal of Physical Medicine & Rehabilitation, 82(5), 338–344.*

Bolgla, L. A., & Uhl, T. L. (2007). Reliability of electromyographic normalization methods for evaluating the hip musculature. *Journal of Electromyography and Kinesiology, 17(1), 102–111.*

Bouchard, C., Shephard, R. J., Stephens, T., Sutton, J. R., & McPherson, B. D. (1990). Proceedings from ICEFH '90: *The International Conference on Exercise, Fitness, and Health. Toronto: Canada.*

Bronfort, G., Goldsmith, C. H., Nelson, C. F., Boline, P. D., & Anderson, A. V. (1995). Trunk exercise combined with spinal manipulative or NSAID therapy for chronic low back pain: a randomized, observer-blinded clinical trial. *Journal of Manipulative and Physiological Therapeutics, 19 (9) 570-582.*

Byström, M. G., Rasmussen-Barr, E., & Grooten, W. J. A. (2013). Motor control exercises reduces pain and disability in chronic and recurrent low back pain: a meta-analysis. *Spine, 38(6), E350-E358.*

Cady, L. D., Bischoff, D. P., O'connell, E. R., Thomas, P. C., & Allan, J. H. (1979). Strength and fitness and subsequent back injuries in firefighters. *Journal of Occupational and Environmental Medicine, 21(4) 269-272.*

Cairns, M. C., Foster, N. E., & Wright, C. (2006). Randomized controlled trial of specific spinal stabilization exercises and conventional physiotherapy for recurrent low back pain. *Spine, 31(19), E670-E681.*

Callaghan, J. P., Gunning, J. L., & McGill, S. M. (1998). The relationship between lumbar spine load and muscle activity during extensor exercises. *Physical therapy, 78(1), 8.*

Carey, T. S., Evans, A. T., Hadler, N. M., Lieberman, G., Kalsbeek, W. D., Jackman, A. M., ... & McNutt, R. A. (1996). Acute severe low back pain: a population-based study of prevalence and care-seeking. *Spine, 21 (3) 339-344.*

Carrera-Bastos, P., Fontes-Villalba, M., O'Keefe, J. H., Lindeberg, S., & Cordain, L. (2011). The western diet and lifestyle and diseases of civilization. *Research Reports in Clinical Cardiology, 2, 15–35.*

Centers for Disease Control and Prevention (CDC. (2001). Prevalence of disabilities and associated health conditions among adults--United States, 1999. MMWR. *Morbidity and Mortality Weekly Report, 50 (7) 120.*

Cerrah, A. O., Ertan, H., & Soylu, A. R. (2010). Spor bilimlerinde elektromiyografi kullanımı. *Spormetre Beden Eğitimi ve Spor Bilimleri Dergisi, 8(2), 43–49.*

Chaiamnuay, P., Darmawan, J., Muirden, K. D., & Assawatanabodee, P. (1998). Epidemiology of rheumatic disease in rural Thailand: A who-Ilar Copcord study. *The Journal of Rheumatology, 25 (7) 1382-1387.*

Chok, B., Lee, R., Latimer, J., & Tan, S. B. (1999). Endurance training of the trunk extensor muscles in people with subacute low back pain. *Physical Therapy, 79 (11) 1032.*

Cholewicki, J., & McGill, S. M. (1996). Mechanical stability of the in vivo lumbar spine: implications for injury and chronic low back pain. *Clinical biomechanics, 11(1), 1-15.*

Chou, R., & Huffman, L. H. (2007). Medications for Acute and Chronic Low Back Pain: A Review of the Evidence for an American Pain Society/American College of Physicians Clinical Practice GuidelineMedications for Acute and Chronic Low Back Pain. *Annals of Internal Medicine, 147(7), 505–514.*

Chou, R., Qaseem, A., Snow, V., Casey, D., Cross, J. T., Shekelle, P., & Owens, D. K. (2007). Diagnosis and Treatment of Low Back Pain: A Joint Clinical Practice Guideline from the American College of Physicians and the American Pain SocietyDiagnosis and Treatment of Low Back Pain. *Annals of Internal Medicine, 147(7), 478–491.*

Clarys, J. P. (2000). Electromyography in sports and occupational settings: *an update of its limits and possibilities. Ergonomics, 43(10), 1750–1762.*

Clarys, J. P., Scafoglieri, A., Tresignie, J., Reilly, T., & Van Roy, P. (2010). Critical appraisal and hazards of surface electromyography data acquisition in sport and exercise. *Asian Journal of Sports Medicine, 1(2), 69.*

Contreras, B., & Schoenfeld, B. (2011). To crunch or not to crunch: An evidence-based examination of spinal flexion exercises, their potential risks, and their applicability to program design. *Strength & Conditioning Journal, 33 (4) 8-18.*

Cooper, N. A., Tipayamongkol, N., Scavo, K. M., Strickland, K. J., Nicholson, J. D., Bewyer, D. C., & Sluka, K. (2013). Prevalence Of Gluteus Medius Weakness In People With Low Back Pain Compared To Age-And Sex-matched Controls Without Low Back Pain. *Journal of Orthopaedic & Sports Physical, 43(1), A75–A76.*

Cordova, M. L., Ingersoll, C. D., Kovaleski, J. E., & Knight, K. L. (1995). A comparison of isokinetic and isotonic predictions of a functional task. *Journal of Athletic Training, 30 (4) 319.*

Council, N. R. (2001). Musculoskeletal disorders and the workplace: low back and upper extremities. *National Academies Press.*

Cram, J. R. (1998). Introduction to surface electromyography. *Aspen Publishers.*

Cresswell, A. G., Oddsson, L., & Thorstensson, A. (1994). The influence of sudden perturbations on trunk muscle activity and intra-abdominal pressure while standing. *Experimental Brain Research, 98(2), 336–341.*

Criswell, E. (2010). Cram's Introduction to Surface Electromyography. *Jones & Bartlett Publishers.*

Croft, P. R., Macfarlane, G. J., Papageorgiou, A. C., Thomas, E., & Silman, A. J. (1998). *Outcome of low back pain in general practice: a prospective study. Bmj, 316(7141), 1356.*

Daerga, L., Edin-Liljegren, A., & Sjölander, P. (2004). Work-related musculoskeletal pain among reindeer herding Sami in Sweden-a pilot study on causes and prevention. *International Journal of Circumpolar Health, 63(sup2), 343–348.*

Dagenais, S., Caro, J., & Haldeman, S. (2008). A systematic review of low back pain cost of illness studies in the United States and internationally. *The Spine Journal, 8(1), 8–20.*

Damasceno, L. H. F., Catarin, S. R. G., Campos, A. D., & Defino, H. L. A. (2006). Lumbar lordosis: a study of angle values and of vertebral bodies and intervertebral discs role. *Acta Ortopédica Brasileira, 14 (4) 193-198.*

Danneels, L. A., Cagnie, B. J., Cools, A. M., Vanderstraeten, G. G., Cambier, D. C., Witvrouw, E. E., & De Cuyper, H. J. (2001). Intra-operator and inter-operator reliability of surface electromyography in the clinical evaluation of back muscles. *Manual Therapy, 6(3), 145–153.*

Danneels, L. A., Vanderstraeten, G. G., Cambier, D. C., Witvrouw, E. E., Bourgois, J. D. W. D. C. H. J., Dankaerts, W., & De Cuyper, H. J. (2001). Effects of three different training modalities on the cross sectional area of the lumbar multifidus muscle in patients with chronic low back pain. *British Journal of Sports Medicine, 35 (3) 186-191.*

Danneels, L. A., Vanderstraeten, G. G., Cambier, D. C., Witvrouw, E. E., De Cuyper, H. J., & Danneels, L. (2000). CT imaging of trunk muscles in chronic low back pain patients and healthy control subjects. *European Spine Journal, 9(4), 266–272.*

Danneels, L., Coorevits, P., Cools, A., Vanderstraeten, G., Cambier, D., Witvrouw, E., & De Cuyper, H. (2002). Differences in electromyographic activity in the multifidus muscle and the iliocostalis lumborum between healthy subjects and patients with sub-acute and chronic low back pain. *European Spine Journal, 11 (1) 13-19.*

Davidson, K. L. C., & Hubley-Kozey, C. L. (2005). Trunk muscle responses to demands of an exercise progression to improve dynamic spinal stability. *Archives of Physical Medicine and Rehabilitation, 86 (2) 216-223.*

De Luca, C. J. (1997). The use of surface electromyography in biomechanics. *Journal of Applied Biomechanics, 13(2), 135–163.*

Delitto, A., Erhard, R. E., & Bowling, R. W. (1995). A treatment-based classification approach to low back syndrome: identifying and staging patients for conservative treatment. *Physical therapy, 75(6), 470-85.*

Deluca, C. J. (2010). *"Surface electromyography: detection and recording"2002. DelSys Inc.(Cited on Page 39.).*

Deyo, R. A. (1996). Drug therapy for back pain: which drugs help which patients? *Spine, 21(24), 2840–2849.*

Deyo, R. A., & Bass, J. E. (1989). Lifestyle and low-back pain: the influence of smoking and obesity. *Spine, 14(5), 501–506.*

Distefano, L. J., Blackburn, J. T., Marshall, S. W., & Padua, D. A. (2009). Gluteal muscle activation during common therapeutic exercises. *Journal of Orthopaedic & Sports Physical Therapy, 39 (7) 532-540.*

Donelson, R., McIntosh, G., & Hall, H. (2012). Is it time to rethink the typical course of low back pain? *PM&R, 4(6), 394–401.*

Donner, A., & Klar, N. (2004). Pitfalls of and controversies in cluster randomization trials. *American Journal of Public Health, 94(3),* *416-422.*

Draper, N., & Hodgson, C. (2008). *Adventure sport physiology. John Wiley & Sons.*

Duthey, B. (2013). *Background Paper 6.24 Low back pain.*

Ebrahimi, H., Blaouchi, R., Eslami, R., & Shahrokhi, M. (2014). Effect of 8-week core stabilization exercises on low back pain, abdominal and back muscle endurance in patients with chronic low back pain due to disc herniation. *Physical Treatments-Specific Physical Therapy Journal, 4 (1) 25-32.*

Ebrahimi, I., Shah Hosseini, G. R., Farahini, H., & Arab, A. (2005). Clinical trunk muscle endurance tests in subjects with and without low back pain. *Medical Journal of The Islamic Republic of Iran (MJIRI), 19 (2) 95-101.*

Edmonds, M., McGuire, H., & Price, J. (2004). Exercise therapy for chronic fatigue syndrome. *Cochrane Database Syst Rev, 3.*

Ekman, M., Johnell, O., & Lidgren, L. (2005). The economic cost of low back pain in Sweden in 2001. *Acta Orthopaedica, 76(2), 275–284.*

Ekstrom, R. A., Donatelli, R. A., & Carp, K. C. (2007). Electromyographic analysis of core trunk, hip, and thigh muscles during 9 rehabilitation exercises. *Journal of Orthopaedic & Sports Physical Therapy, 37(12), 754–762.*

Ekstrom, R. A., Osborn, R. W., & Hauer, P. L. (2008). Surface electromyographic analysis of the low back muscles during rehabilitation exercises. *Journal of Orthopaedic & Sports Physical Therapy, 38 (12) 736-745.*

Ellis, P. D. (2010). *The essential guide to effect sizes: Statistical power, meta analysis, and the interpretation of research results. Cambridge University Press.*

Escamilla, R. F., Babb, E., DeWitt, R., & Jew, P. (2006). Electromyographic analysis of traditional and nontraditional abdominal exercises: *implications for rehabilitation and training. Physical Therapy, 86 (5) 656.*

Evans, G., & Richards, S. (1996). Low back pain: an evaluation of therapeutic interventions. *Health Care Evaluation Unit, University of Bristol Bristol.*

Faas, A. (1996). Exercises: which ones are worth trying, for which patients, and when?. *Spine, 21 (24) 2874-2878.*

Fahey, T., Insel, P., & Roth, W. (2012). Fit & Well Alternate Edition: Core Concepts and Labs in Physical Fitness and Wellness. *McGraw-Hill Higher Education.*

Fast, A., Weiss, L., Ducommun, E. J., Medina, E., & Butler, J. G. (1990). Low-Back Pain in Pregnancy Abdominal Muscles, Sit-up Performance, and Back Pain. *Spine, 15(1), 28–30.*

Fauth, M. L., Petushek, E. J., Feldmann, C. R., Hsu, B. E., Garceau, L. R., Lutsch, B. N., & Ebben, W. P. (2010). Reliability of surface electromyography during maximal voluntary isometric contractions, jump landings, and cutting. *The Journal of Strength & Conditioning Research, 24(4), 1131–1137.*

Ferreira, M. L., Ferreira, P. H., Latimer, J., Herbert, R. D., Hodges, P. W., Jennings, M. D., & Refshauge, K. M. (2007). Comparison of general exercise, motor control exercise and spinal manipulative therapy for chronic low back pain: a randomized trial. *Pain, 131(1), 31-37.*

Foster, N. E., Thompson, K. A., Baxter, G. D., & Allen, J. M. (1999). Management of nonspecific low back pain by physiotherapists in Britain and Ireland: a descriptive questionnaire of current clinical practice. *Spine, 24(13), 1332.*

França, F. R., Burke, T. N., Hanada, E. S., & Marques, A. P. (2010). Segmental stabilization and muscular strengthening in chronic low back pain: a comparative study. *Clinics, 65 (10) 1013-1017.*

Freburger, J. K., Holmes, G. M., Agans, R. P., Jackman, A. M., Darter, J. D., Wallace, A. S., … Carey, T. S. (2009). The rising prevalence of chronic low back pain. *Archives of Internal Medicine, 169(3), 251–258.*

Frymoyer, J. W. (1988). Back pain and sciatica. *New England Journal of Medicine, 318(5), 291–300.*

Garcia, A. N., Costa, L. D. C. M., da Silva, T. M., Gondo, F. L. B., Cyrillo, F. N., Costa, R. A., & Costa, L. O. P. (2013). Effectiveness of back school versus McKenzie exercises in patients with chronic nonspecific low back pain: a randomized controlled trial. *Physical Therapy, 93 (6) 729.*

Garcia, M. A. C., & Vieira, T. M. M. (2011). Surface electromyography: Why, when and how to use it. *Revista Andaluza de Medicina Del Deporte, 4(1), 17–28.*

Gardner-Morse, M., Stokes, I. A., & Laible, J. P. (1995). Role of muscles in lumbar spine stability in maximum extension efforts. *Journal of Orthopaedic Research, 13(5), 802-808.*

Geddes, L. A. (1972). *Electrodes and the measurement of bioelectric events Wiley. New York, NY.*

Gracovetsky, S. (2010). Non Invasive Assessment of Spinal Function. Automatizing the Physical Examination. Canada: *Aardvark Global Publishing.*

Grieve, G. P. (1982). Lumbar instability. *Physiotherapy, 68(1), 2.*

Group, T. W. (1998). The World Health Organization quality of life assessment (WHOQOL): development and general psychometric properties. *Social Science & Medicine, 46(12), 1569–1585.*

Guo, H. R., Tanaka, S., Halperin, W. E., & Cameron, L. L. (1999). Back pain prevalence in US industry and estimates of lost workdays. *American Journal of Public Health, 89 (7) 1029-1035.*

Halldin, K., Zoega, B., Kärrholm, J., Lind, B. I., & Nyberg, P. (2005). Is increased segmental motion early after lumbar discectomy related to poor clinical outcome 5 years later? *International Orthopaedics, 29(4), 260–264.*

Hayden, J. A., Van Tulder, M. W., Malmivaara, A. V., & Koes, B. W. (2005). Meta-analysis: exercise therapy for nonspecific low back pain. *Annals of Internal Medicine, 142 (9) 765-775.*

Hazard, R. G., Fenwick, J. W., Kalisch, S. M., Redmond, J., Reeves, V., Reid, S., & Frymoyer, J. W. (1989). Functional Restoration with Behavioral

Support: A One-Year Prospective Study of Patients with Chronic Low-Back Pain. *Spine, 14(2), 157–161.*

Heeren, T., & D›Agostino, R. (1987). Robustness of the two independent samples t-test when applied to ordinal scaled data. *Statistics in medicine, 6(1), 79-90.*

Helmhout, P. H., Staal, J. B., Maher, C. G., Petersen, T., Rainville, J., & Shaw, W. S. (2008). Exercise therapy and low back pain: insights and proposals to improve the design, conduct, and reporting of clinical trials. *Spine, 33 (16) 1782-1788.*

Hendrick, P., Milosavljevic, S., Hale, L., Hurley, D. A., McDonough, S., Ryan, B., & Baxter, G. D. (2011). The relationship between physical activity and low back pain outcomes: a systematic review of observational studies. *European Spine Journal, 20(3), 464–474.*

Hendrix, C. R., Housh, T. J., Johnson, G. O., Mielke, M., Camic, C. L., Zuniga, J. M., & Schmidt, R. J. (2009). Comparison of critical force to EMG fatigue thresholds during isometric leg extension. *Medicine & Science in Sports & Exercise, 41(4), 956–964.*

Hicks, G. E., Fritz, J. M., Delitto, A., & McGill, S. M. (2005). Preliminary development of a clinical prediction rule for determining which patients with low back pain will respond to a stabilization exercise program. *Archives of Physical Medicine and Rehabilitation, 86(9), 1753–1762.*

Hides, J. A., Jull, G. A., & Richardson, C. A. (2001). Long-term effects of specific stabilizing exercises for first-episode low back pain. *Spine, 26(11), e243-e248.*

Hides, J. A., Richardson, C. A., & Jull, G. A. (1996). Multifidus Muscle Recovery Is Not Automatic After Resolution of Acute, First-Episode Low Back Pain. *Spine, 21(23), 2763-2769.*

Hintermeister, R. A., Lange, G. W., Schultheis, J. M., Bey, M. J., & Hawkins, R. J. (1998). Electromyographic activity and applied load during shoulder rehabilitation exercises using elastic resistance. *The American Journal of Sports Medicine, 26(2), 210–220.*

Hodges, P. W. (1999). Is there a role for transversus abdominis in lumbo-pelvic stability?. *Manual therapy, 4(2), 74-86.*

Hodges, P. W., & Richardson, C. A. (1997). Feedforward contraction of transversus abdominis is not influenced by the direction of arm movement. *Experimental Brain Research, 114(2), 362–370.*

Hodges, P. W., & Richardson, C. A. (1998). Delayed postural contraction of transversus abdominis in low back pain associated with movement of the lower limb. *Clinical Spine Surgery, 11(1), 46–56.*

Hodges, P. W., & Richardson, C. A. (1999). Transversus abdominis and the superficial abdominal muscles are controlled independently in a postural task. *Neuroscience Letters, 265(2), 91–94.*

Hodges, P. W., & Smeets, R. J. (2015). Interaction between pain, movement, and physical activity: short-term benefits, long-term consequences, and targets for treatment. *The Clinical Journal of Pain, 31(2), 97–107.*

Hoff, J., & Helgerud, J. (2004). Endurance and strength training for soccer players. *Sports Medicine, 34(3), 165–180.*

Holmes, B., Leggett, S., Mooney, V., Nichols, J., Negri, S., & Hoeyberghs, A. (1996). Comparison of female geriatric lumbar-extension strength:

asymptotic versus chronic low back pain patients and their response to active rehabilitation. *Clinical Spine Surgery, 9(1), 17–22.*

Honeyman, P. T., & Jacobs, E. A. (1996). Effects of culture on back pain in Australian aboriginals. *Spine, 21(7), 841–843.*

Hosseinifar, M., Akbari, M., Behtash, H., Amiri, M., & Sarrafzadeh, J. (2013). The effects of stabilization and McKenzie exercises on transverse abdominis and multifidus muscle thickness, pain, and disability: a randomized controlled trial in nonspecific chronic low back pain. *Journal of Physical Therapy Science, 25 (12) 1541-1545.*

Hoy, D., Brooks, P., Blyth, F., & Buchbinder, R. (2010). The epidemiology of low back pain. *Best Practice & Research Clinical Rheumatology, 24 (6) 769-781.*

Hurwitz, E. L., Morgenstern, H., & Chiao, C. (2005). Effects of recreational physical activity and back exercises on low back pain and psychological distress: findings from the UCLA Low Back Pain Study. *American Journal of Public Health, 95(10), 1817–1824.*

Hussain, I., & Sharma, K. (2008). Electromyographic comparison of abdominal muscle activation during Sit-Up exercise and Ab crunch. *International Journal of Sports Science and Engineering, World Academic Union.*

Illyés, Á., & Kiss, R. M. (2005). Shoulder muscle activity during pushing, pulling, elevation and overhead throw. *Journal of Electromyography and Kinesiology, 15(3), 282–289.*

Ingersoll, C. D., & Knight, K. L. (1991). Patellar location changes following EMG biofeedback or progressive resistive exercises. *Medicine and Science in Sports and Exercise, 23 (10) 1122-1127.*

Jackson, C. P., & Brown, M. D. (1983). Is There a Role for Exercise in the Treatment of Patients with Low Back Pain?. *Clinical Orthopaedics and Related Research, 179, 39-45.*

Jenkins, G., & Tortora, G. J. (2011). *Anatomy and physiology. Wiley-Blackwell.*

John, P. J., Sharma, N., Sharma, C. M., & Kankane, A. (2007). Effectiveness of yoga therapy in the treatment of migraine without aura: a randomized controlled trial. *Headache: The Journal of Head and Face Pain 47 (5) 654-661.*

Kaltenborn, F. M. (1970). Mobilization of the spinal column. *New Zealand University Press.*

Kamaz, M., Kiresi, D., Oguz, H., Emlik, D., & Levendoglu, F. (2007). CT measurement of trunk muscle areas in patients with chronic low back pain. *Diagnostic and Interventional Radiology, 13(3), 144.*

Kankaanpää, M., Taimela, S., Laaksonen, D., Hänninen, O., & Airaksinen, O. (1998). Back and hip extensor fatigability in chronic low back pain patients and controls. *Archives of Physical Medicine and Rehabilitation, 79(4), 412–417.*

Karmisholt, K., & Gotzsche, P. (2005). Physical activity for secondary prevention of disease. *Dan Med Bull, 52(2), 90–94.*

Karşılaştırılması, E. P. (2014). *Efficacy of core-stabilization exercise and its comparison with home-based conventional exercise in low back pain patients.*

Karunanayake, A. L., Pathmeswaran, A., Kasturiratne, A., & Wijeyaratne, L. S. (2013). Risk factors for chronic low back pain in a sample of suburban Sri Lankan adult males. *International Journal of Rheumatic Diseases, 16 (2) 203-210.*

Katirji, B. (2007). Electromyography in Clinical Practice E-Book: A Case Study Approach. *Elsevier Health Sciences.*

Katz, J. N. (2006). Lumbar disc disorders and low-back pain: socioeconomic factors and consequences. *JBJS, 88(suppl_2), 21–24.*

Kellett, K. M., Kellett, D. A., & Nordholm, L. A. (1991). Effects of an exercise program on sick leave due to back pain. *Physical Therapy, 71(4), 283–291.*

Kellis, E., & Katis, A. (2008). Reliability of EMG power-spectrum and amplitude of the semitendinosus and biceps femoris muscles during ramp isometric contractions. *Journal of Electromyography and Kinesiology, 18(3), 351–358.*

Kelsey, J. L., Githens, P. B., O'conner, T., Weil, U., Calogero, J. A., Holford, T. R., ... Southwick, W. O. (1984). Acute Prolapsed Lumbar Intervertebral Disc An Epidemiologic Study with Special Reference to Driving Automobiles and Cigarette Smoking. *Spine, 9(6), 608–613.*

Kendall FP, McCreary EK, Provance PG, Rodgers MM, Romani WA. (2005). Muscles: Testing and Function With Posture and Pain. *Baltimore, MD: Lippincott, Williams & Wilkins.*

Kent, P. M., & Keating, J. L. (2008). Can we predict poor recovery from recent-onset nonspecific low back pain? A systematic review. *Manual Therapy, 13(1), 12–28.*

Khan, A. A., Uddin, M. M., Chowdhury, A. H., & Guha, R. K. (2014). Association of low back pain with common risk factors: a community based study. *Indian J Med Res, 25, 50-55.*

Kibler, W. B., Press, J., & Sciascia, A. (2006). The role of core stability in athletic function. *Sports Medicine, 36 (3) 189-198.*

Koes, B. W., Bouter, L. M., & van der Heijden, G. J. M. G. (1995). Methodological Quality of Randomized Clinical Trials on Treatment Efficcact in Low Back Pain. *Spine, 20(2), 228–235.*

Koes, B. W., van Tulder, M. W., Ostelo, R., Burton, A. K., & Waddell, G. (2001). Clinical guidelines for the management of low back pain in primary care: an international comparison. *Spine, 26(22), 2504–2513.*

Kool, J., de Bie, R. A., Oesch, P., Knusel, O., van den Brandt, P. A., & Bachmann, S. (2004). *Exercise reduces sick leave in patients with non-acute non-specific low back pain: a meta-analysis.*

Koumantakis, G. A., Watson, P. J., & Oldham, J. A. (2005). Trunk muscle stabilization training plus general exercise versus general exercise only: randomized controlled trial of patients with recurrent low back pain. *Physical Therapy, 85 (3) 209.*

Lamontagne, M. (2002). Application of Electromyography in Movement Studies. *International Research in Sports Biomechanics, 137.*

Lamoth, C. J. C., Meijer, O. G., Wuisman, P. I. J. M., van Dieën, J. H., Levin, M. F., & Beek, P. J. (2002). Pelvis-thorax coordination in the transverse plane during walking in persons with nonspecific low back pain. *Spine, 27(4), E92–E99.*

Lamoth, C. J. C., Stins, J. F., Pont, M., Kerckhoff, F., & Beek, P. J. (2008). Effects of attention on the control of locomotion in individuals with chronic low back pain. *Journal of Neuroengineering and Rehabilitation, 5(1), 13.*

Langevin, H. M., & Sherman, K. J. (2007). Pathophysiological model for chronic low back pain integrating connective tissue and nervous system mechanisms. *Medical Hypotheses, 68(1), 74–80.*

Lawrence, J. H., & De Luca, C. J. (1983). Myoelectric signal versus force relationship in different human muscles. *Journal of Applied Physiology, 54(6), 1653–1659.*

Lee, G. K., Chronister, J., & Bishop, M. (2008). The effects of psychosocial factors on quality of life among individuals with chronic pain. *Rehabilitation Counseling Bulletin.*

Lee, J.-H., Hoshino, Y., Nakamura, K., Kariya, Y., Saita, K., & Ito, K. (1999). Trunk Muscle Weakness as a Risk Factor for Low Back Pain: A 5-Year Prospective Study. *Spine, 24(1), 54–57.*

Leetun, D. T., Ireland, M. L., Willson, J. D., Ballantyne, B. T., & Davis, I. M. (2004). Core stability measures as risk factors for lower extremity injury in athletes. *Medicine & Science in Sports & Exercise, 36(6), 926–934.*

Leinonen, V., Kankaanpää, M., Airaksinen, O., & Hänninen, O. (2000). Back and hip extensor activities during trunk flexion/extension: effects of low back pain and rehabilitation. *Archives of Physical Medicine and Rehabilitation, 81(1), 32–37.*

Lewis, A., Morris, M. E., & Walsh, C. (2008). Are physiotherapy exercises effective in reducing chronic low back pain? *Physical Therapy Reviews, 13(1), 37–44.*

Liddle, S. D., Gracey, J. H., & Baxter, G. D. (2007). Advice for the management of low back pain: a systematic review of randomised controlled trials. *Manual Therapy, 12(4), 310–327.*

Lieber, R. L., & Fridén, J. (2002). Morphologic and mechanical basis of delayed-onset muscle soreness. *Journal of the American Academy of Orthopaedic Surgeons, 10(1), 67–73.*

Lindeberg, S., Cordain, L., & Eaton, S. B. (2003). Biological and clinical potential of a palaeolithic diet. *Journal of Nutritional & Environmental Medicine, 13(3), 149–160.*

Luque-Suárez, A., Díaz-Mohedo, E., Medina-Porqueres, I., & Ponce-García, T. (2012). Stabilization exercise for the management of low back pain. *INTECH Open Access Publisher.*

Macedo, L. G., Bostick, G. P., & Maher, C. G. (2013). Exercise for prevention of recurrences of nonspecific low back pain. *Physical Therapy, 93(12), 1587–1591.*

Machado, L. A. C., De Souza, M. V. S., Ferreira, P. H., & Ferreira, M. L. (2006). The McKenzie method for low back pain: a systematic review of the literature with a meta-analysis approach. *Spine, 31 (9) 254-262.*

MacIsaac, D., Parker, P. A., & Scott, R. N. (2001). The short-time Fourier transform and muscle fatigue assessment in dynamic contractions. *Journal of Electromyography and Kinesiology, 11(6), 439–449.*

Maitland, G. D. (2005). *Maitland's vertebral manipulation (Vol. 1)*. *Butterworth-Heinemann*.

Majid, K., & Truumees, E. (2008). Epidemiology and natural history of low back pain. *In Seminars in Spine Surgery (Vol. 20, pp. 87–92). Elsevier.*

Malmivaara, A., Häkkinen, U., Aro, T., Heinrichs, M.-L., Koskenniemi, L., Kuosma, E., ... Vaaranen, V. (1995). The treatment of acute low back pain—bed rest, exercises, or ordinary activity? *New England Journal of Medicine, 332(6), 351–355.*

Mamashli, S., Mahdavinejad, R., & Goodarzi, B. (2014). The Comparison of the Effect of Eight Weeks of Pilates and Stabilization Exercises on Pain and Functional Disability of Women with Chronic Low Back Pain. *European academic research, 1(10), 3373-3384.*

Maniadakis, N., & Gray, A. (2000). The economic burden of back pain in the UK. *Pain, 84(1), 95–103.*

Mannion, A. F., Adams, M. A., Cooper, R. G., & Dolan, P. (1999). Prediction of maximal back muscle strength from indices of body mass and fat-free body mass. *Rheumatology (Oxford, England), 38(7), 652–655.*

Mannion, A. F., Müntener, M., Taimela, S., & Dvorak, J. (2001). Comparison of three active therapies for chronic low back pain: results of a randomized clinical trial with one-year follow-up. *Rheumatology, 40 (7) 772-778.*

Marras, W. S., Rangarajulu, S. L., & Lavender, S. A. (1987). Trunk loading and expectation. *Ergonomics, 30 (3) 551-562.*

Martin, C. K., Church, T. S., Thompson, A. M., Earnest, C. P., & Blair, S. N. (2009). Exercise dose and quality of life: a randomized controlled trial. *Archives of Internal Medicine, 169(3), 269–278.*

Massó, N., Rey, F., Romero, D., Gual, G., Costa, L., & Germán, A. (2010). Surface electromyography applications. *Apunts Medicina de l» Esport (English Edition), 45(166), 127–136.*

May, A. M., Van Weert, E., Korstjens, I., Hoekstra-Weebers, J. E. H. M., Van Der Schans, C. P., Zonderland, M. L., ... Ros, W. J. G. (2008). Improved physical fitness of cancer survivors: a randomised controlled trial comparing physical training with physical and cognitive-behavioural training. *Acta Oncologica, 47(5), 825–834.*

May, S., & Johnson, R. (2008). Stabilisation exercises for low back pain: a systematic review. *Physiotherapy, 94(3), 179-189.*

Mayer, T. G., Gatchel, R. J., KisHiNo, N., Keeley, J., Capra, P., Mayer, H., ... Mooney, V. (1985). Objective assessment of spine function following industrial injury. A prospective study with comparison group and one-year follow-up. *Spine, 10(6), 482–493.*

Mayer, T. G., Kondraske, G., Mooney, V., Carmichael, T. W., & Butsch, R. (1989). Lumbar Myoelectric Spectral Analysis for Endurance Assessment: A Comparison of Normals with Deconditioned Patients. *Spine, 14(9), 986-991.*

McArdle, W. D., Katch, F. I., & Katch, V. L. (2007). Pulmonary structure and function. Exercise Physiology, 6th Edn. *Williams & Wilkins, Philadelphia, 260–270.*

McCarthy, C. J., Callaghan, M. J., & Oldham, J. A. (2008). The reliability of isometric strength and fatigue measures in patients with knee osteoarthritis. *Manual Therapy, 13(2), 159–164.*

McKenzie, R. A., & May, S. (1981). The lumbar spine. *Mechanical Diagnosis & Therapy, 1, 374.*

Merletti, R., Rainoldi, A., & Farina, D. (2001). Surface electromyography for noninvasive characterization of muscle. *Exercise and Sport Sciences Reviews, 29(1), 20–25.*

Metgud, D. C., Khatri, S., Mokashi, M. G., & Saha, P. N. (2008). An ergonomic study of women workers in a woolen textile factory for identification of health-related problems. *Indian Journal of Occupational and Environmental Medicine, 12 (1) 14.*

Micheli, L. J. (2010). *Encyclopedia of sports medicine (Vol. 3). Sage.*

Moffett, J. K., Richardson, G., Sheldon, T., & Maynard, A. (1995). *Back pain: its management and costs to society.*

Monfort-Pañego, M., Vera-García, F. J., Sánchez-Zuriaga, D., & Sarti-Martínez, M. Á. (2009). Electromyographic studies in abdominal exercises: a literature synthesis. *Journal of Manipulative and Physiological Therapeutics, 32 (3) 232-244.*

Moon, H. J., Choi, K. H., Kim, D. H., Kim, H. J., Cho, Y. K., Lee, K. H., ... & Choi, Y. J. (2013). Effect of lumbar stabilization and dynamic lumbar strengthening exercises in patients with chronic low back pain. Annals of Rehabilitation Medicine, 37 (1) 110-117.

Mooney, V., Gulick, J., Perlman, M., Levy, D., Pozos, R., Leggett, S., & Resnick, D. (1997). Relationships between myoelectric activity, strength, and MRI of lumbar extensor muscles in back pain patients and normal subjects. *Clinical Spine Surgery, 10(4), 348-356.*

Moore, K. L., Dalley, A. F., & Agur, A. M. R. (2013). *Clinically oriented anatomy. Lippincott Williams & Wilkins.*

MORAIS, G. C. (2011). Estrutura das assembléias de macroinvertebrados de substratos rochosos no litoral de Curuçá, nordeste do Pará, Brasil. *Universidade Federal do Pará.*

Morgan, M. H. (1989). Nerve conduction studies. *British Journal of Hospital Medicine, 41(1), 22–26.*

Nachemson, A. (1983). Work for all: for those with low back pain as well. *Clinical Orthopaedics and Related Research, 179, 77–85.*

Nachemson, A., Waddell, G., & Norlund, A. I. (2000). *Epidemiology of neck and low back pain. Neck and Back Pain: The Scientific Evidence of Causes, Diagnosis and Treatment, 165-188.*

Nadler, S. F., Malanga, G. A., Bartoli, L. A., Feinberg, J. H., Prybicien, M., & DePrince, M. (2002). Hip muscle imbalance and low back pain in athletes: influence of core strengthening. *Medicine & Science in Sports & Exercise, 34 (1) 9-16.*

Näyhä, S., Videman, T., Laakso, M., & Hassi, J. (1991). Prevalence of low back pain and other musculoskeletal symptoms and their association with work in Finnish reindeer herders. *Scandinavian Journal of Rheumatology, 20(6), 406–413.*

Norris, C. M. (2008). Back stability: integrating science and therapy. 2nd. ed. Champaign, IL: *Human Kinetics; pp. 9–20.*

Nourbakhsh, M. R., & Arab, A. M. (2002). Relationship between mechanical factors and incidence of low back pain. *Journal of Orthopaedic & Sports Physical Therapy, 32 (9), 447-460.*

Oddsson, L. (1988). Co-ordination of a simple voluntary multi-joint movement with postural demands: Trunk extension in standing man. *Acta Physiologica, 134(1), 109–118.*

Ogawa, T., Matsuzaki, H., Uei, H., Nakajima, S., Tokuhashi, Y., & Esumi, M. (2005). Alteration of gene expression in intervertebral disc degeneration of passive cigarette-smoking rats: separate quantitation in separated nucleus pulposus and annulus fibrosus. *Pathobiology, 72 (3) 146-151.*

Ogon, M., Bender, B. R., Hooper, D. M., Spratt, K. F., Goel, V. K., Wilder, D. G., & Pope, M. H. (1997). A Dynamic Approach to Spinal Instability: Part II: Hesitation and Giving-Way During Interspinal Motion. *Spine, 22(24), 2859-2866.*

Okubo, Y., Kaneoka, K., Imai, A., Shiina, I., Tatsumura, M., Izumi, S., & Miyakawa, S. (2010). Electromyographic analysis of transversus abdominis and lumbar multifidus using wire electrodes during lumbar stabilization exercises. *Journal of Orthopaedic & Sports Physical Therapy, 40 (11) 743-750.*

Oliver, G. D., Stone, A. J., & Plummer, H. (2010). Electromyographic examination of selected muscle activation during isometric core exercises. *Clinical Journal of Sport Medicine, 20 (6) 452-457.*

Oˏsullivan, P. B., Phyty, G. D. M., Twomey, L. T., & Allison, G. T. (1997). Evaluation of specific stabilizing exercise in the treatment of chronic low back pain with radiologic diagnosis of spondylolysis or spondylolisthesis. *Spine, 22(24), 2959-2967.*

Panjabi, M. M., Lydon, C., Vasavada, A., Grab, D., Crisco III, J. J., & Dvorak, J. (1994). On the understanding of clinical instability. *Spine, 19(23), 2642-2650.*

Papageorgiou, A. C., Macfarlane, G. J., Thomas, E., Croft, P. R., Jayson, M. I. V, & Silman, A. J. (1997). Psychosocial Factors in the Workplace-Do They Predict New Episodes of Low Back Pain?: Evidence From the South Manchester Back Pain Study. *Spine, 22(10), 1137–1142.*

Parnianpour, M., Nordin, M., Kahanovitz, N., & Frankel, V. (1988). The triaxial coupling of torque generation of trunk muscles during isometric exertions and the effect of fatiguing isoinertial movements on the motor output and movement patterns. *Spine, 13(9), 982–992.*

Patton, K. T. (2015). Anatomy and physiology. *Elsevier Health Sciences.*

Pavón, A. G., Rodríguez, N. R., & Iglesias, F. G. (2016). Cross-sectional study of adult women with low back pain: Demographic and clinical profile and factors associated with disability. *Fisioterapia, 38(1), 11-19.*

Pedersen, B. K., & Saltin, B. (2006). Evidence for prescribing exercise as therapy in chronic disease. *Scandinavian Journal of Medicine & Science in Sports, 16 (S1) 3-63.*

Petersen, T., Kryger, P., Ekdahl, C., Olsen, S., & Jacobsen, S. (2002). The effect of McKenzie therapy as compared with that of intensive strengthening training for the treatment of patients with subacute or chronic low back pain: a randomized controlled trial. *Spine, 27 (16) 1702-1709.*

Pitcher, M. J., Behm, D. G., & MacKinnon, S. N. (2007). Reliability of electromyographic and force measures during prone isometric back extension in subjects with and without low back pain. *Applied Physiology, Nutrition, and Metabolism, 33(1), 52–60.*

Plattner, K., Baumeister, J., Lamberts, R. P., & Lambert, M. I. (2011). Dissociation in changes in EMG activation during maximal isometric and submaximal low force dynamic contractions after exercise-induced muscle damage. *Journal of Electromyography and Kinesiology, 21(3), 542-550.*

Pollock, M. L., Leggett, S. H., Graves, J. E., Jones, A., Fulton, M., & Cirulli, J. (1989). Effect of resistance training on lumbar extension strength. *The American Journal of Sports Medicine, 17(5), 624–629.*

Ponte, D. J., Jensen, G. J., & Kent, B. E. (1984). A preliminary report on the use of the McKenzie (1981) protocol versus Williams (1995) protocol in the treatment of low back pain. *Journal of Orthopaedic & Sports Physical Therapy, 6 (2) 130-139.*

Potvin, J. R., & Bent, L. R. (1997). A validation of techniques using surface EMG signals from dynamic contractions to quantify muscle fatigue during repetitive tasks. *Journal of Electromyography and Kinesiology, 7(2), 131–139.*

Quach, J. H. (2007). *Surface electromyography: Use, design & technological overview. Paper Diakses Menggunakan Http://www. Google. Com. Pada, 8.*

Rainville, J., Hartigan, C., Martinez, E., Limke, J., Jouve, C., & Finno, M. (2004). Exercise as a treatment for chronic low back pain. *The Spine Journal, 4(1), 106–115.*

Refshauge, K. M., & Maher, C. G. (2006). Low back pain investigations and prognosis: a review. *British Journal of Sports Medicine, 40(6), 494–498.*

Reid, M. (2004). An assessment of health needs of chronic low back pain patients from general practice. *Journal of Health Psychology, 9 (3) 451-462.*

Reiman, M. P., Weisbach, P. C., & Glynn, P. E. (2009). The hip's influence on low back pain: a distal link to a proximal problem. *Journal of Sport Rehabilitation, 18(1), 24–32.*

Ricci, J. A., Stewart, W. F., Chee, E., Leotta, C., Foley, K., & Hochberg, M. C. (2006). Back pain exacerbations and lost productive time costs in United States workers. *Spine, 31 (26) 3052-3060.*

Richardson, C. A., & Jull, G. A. (1995). Muscle control–pain control. What exercises would you prescribe? *Manual Therapy, 1(1), 2–10.*

Richardson, C. A., Jull, G. A., Hodges, P. W., & Hides, J. A. (1999). *Therapeutic exercise for spinal segmental stabilization in low back pain: scientific basis and clinical approach.* Churchill Livingstone.

Richmond, J. (2012). Multi-factorial causative model for back pain management; relating causative factors and mechanisms to injury presentations and designing time-and cost effective treatment thereof. *Medical Hypotheses, 79(2), 232–240.*

Roy, S. H., De Luca, C. J., Emley, M., & Buijs, R. J. (1995). Spectral Electromyographic Assessment of Back Muscles in Patients With Low Back Muscles in Patients With Low Back Pain Undergoing Rehabilitation. *Spine, 20(1), 38-48.*

Royal College of General Practitioners. (1999). Clinical Guidelines for the Management of Acute Low Back Pain: Clinical Guidelines and Evidence Review. *Royal College of General Practitioners.*

Rubin, D. I. (2007). Epidemiology and risk factors for spine pain. *Neurologic Clinics, 25 (2) 353-371.*

Russell, D., Hoare, Z. S. J., Whitaker, R. H., Whitaker, C. J., & Russell, I. T. (2011). Generalized method for adaptive randomization in clinical trials. *Statistics in Medicine, 30(9), 922-934.*

Sarti, M. A., Monfort, M., Fuster, M. A., & Villaplana, L. A. (1996). Muscle activity in upper and lower rectus abdominus during abdominal exercises. *Archives of Physical Medicine and Rehabilitation, 77 (12) 1293-1297.*

Savigny, P., Kuntze, S., Watson, P., Underwood, M., Ritchie, G., Cotterell, M., ... Coffey, P. (2009). Low back pain: early management of persistent non-specific low back pain. *London: National Collaborating Centre for Primary Care and Royal College of General Practitioners, 14.*

Selkowitz, D. M., Beneck, G. J., & Powers, C. M. (2013). Which exercises target the gluteal muscles while minimizing activation of the tensor fascia lata? Electromyographic assessment using fine-wire electrodes. *Journal of Orthopaedic & Sports Physical Therapy, 43 (2) 54-64.*

Serner, A., Jakobsen, M. D., Andersen, L. L., Hölmich, P., Sundstrup, E., & Thorborg, K. (2013). EMG evaluation of hip adduction exercises for soccer players: implications for exercise selection in prevention and treatment of groin injuries. *British journal of sports medicine, bjsports.*

Shambrook, J., McNee, P., Harris, E. C., Kim, M., Sampson, M., Palmer, K. T., & Coggon, D. (2011). Clinical presentation of low back pain and association with risk factors according to findings on magnetic resonance imaging. *PAIN®, 152(7), 1659–1665.*

Sherman, K. J., Cherkin, D. C., Erro, J., Miglioretti, D. L., & Deyo, R. A. (2005). Comparing Yoga, Exercise, and a Self-Care Book for Chronic Low Back Pain A Randomized, Controlled Trial. *Annals of Internal Medicine, 143 (12) 849-856.*

Sherman, K. J., Cherkin, D. C., Wellman, R. D., Cook, A. J., Hawkes, R. J., Delaney, K., & Deyo, R. A. (2011). A randomized trial comparing yoga, stretching, and a self-care book for chronic low back pain. *Archives of Internal Medicine, 171 (22) 2019-2026.*

Shiple, B. J., & DiNubile, N. A. (1997). Treating low-back pain: Exercise knowns and unknowns. *The Physician and sportsmedicine, 25 (8) 51-66.*

Slade, S. C., & Keating, J. L. (2006). Trunk-strengthening exercises for chronic low back pain: a systematic review. *Journal of Manipulative and Physiological Therapeutics, 29 (2) 163-173.*

Smith, N. (1999). Gluteus medius function and low back pain; is there a relationship? *Physical Therapy Reviews, 4(4), 283–288.*

Soderberg, G. L., & Knutson, L. M. (2000). A guide for use and interpretation of kinesiologic electromyographic data. *Physical Therapy, 80(5), 485–498.*

Sozen, H. (2010). Comparison of muscle activation during elliptical trainer, treadmill and bike exercise. *Biology of Sport, 27(3), 203.*

Standaert, C. J., Weinstein, S. M., & Rumpeltes, J. (2008). Evidence-informed management of chronic low back pain with lumbar stabilization exercises. *The Spine Journal, 8(1), 114–120.*

Steele, C. M., Bennett, J. W., Chapman-Jay, S., Polacco, R. C., Molfenter, S. M., & Oshalla, M. (2012). Electromyography as a biofeedback tool for rehabilitating swallowing muscle function. *In Applications of EMG in Clinical and Sports Medicine. InTech.*

Steenstra, I. A., Anema, J. R., Bongers, P. M., De Vet, H. C. W., Knol, D. L., & van Mechelen, W. (2006). The effectiveness of graded activity for low back pain in occupational healthcare. *Occupational and Environmental Medicine, 63(11), 718–725.*

Stevens, V. K., Vleeming, A., Bouche, K. G., Mahieu, N. N., Vanderstraeten, G. G., & Danneels, L. A. (2007). Electromyographic activity of trunk and hip muscles during stabilization exercises in four-point kneeling in healthy volunteers. *European Spine Journal, 16 (5) 711-718.*

Stewart, W. F., Ricci, J. A., Chee, E., Morganstein, D., & Lipton, R. (2003). Lost productive time and cost due to common pain conditions in the US workforce. *Jama, 290 (18) 2443-2454.*

Stokes, I. A. F., & Frymoyer, J. W. (1987). Segmental motion and instability. *Spine, 12(7), 688–691.*

Stone, W. J., & Coulter, S. P. (1994). Strength/Endurance Effects From Three Resistance Training Protocols With Women. *The Journal of Strength & Conditioning Research, 8 (4) 231-234.*

Storro, S., Moen, J., & Svebak, S. (2004). Effects on sick-leave of a multidisciplinary rehabilitation programme for chronic low back, neck or shoulder pain: comparison with usual treatment. *Journal of Rehabilitation Medicine, 36(1), 12–16.*

Sutherland, D. H. (2001). The evolution of clinical gait analysis part l: kinesiological EMG. *Gait & Posture, 14(1), 61–70.*

Taimela, S., Kujala, U. M., Salminen, J. J., & Viljanen, T. (1997). The Prevalence of Low Back Pain Among Children and Adolescents: A Nationwide, Cohort-Based Questionnaire Survey in Finland. *Spine, 22(10), 1132–1136.*

Tekur, P., Singphow, C., Nagendra, H. R., & Raghuram, N. (2008). Effect of short-term intensive yoga program on pain, functional disability and spinal flexibility in chronic low back pain: a randomized control study. *The Journal of Alternative and Complementary Medicine, 14 (6) 637-644.*

Tesch, P. A., & Larsson, L. (1982). Muscle hypertrophy in bodybuilders. *European Journal of Applied Physiology and Occupational Physiology, 49(3), 301–306.*

Teyhen, D. S., Rieger, J. L., Westrick, R. B., Miller, A. C., Molloy, J. M., & Childs, J. D. (2008). Changes in deep abdominal muscle thickness during common trunk-strengthening exercises using ultrasound imaging. *Journal of Orthopaedic & Sports Physical Therapy 38(10) 596-605.*

Tomita, S., Arphorn, S., Takashi, M. U. T. O., Koetkhlai, K., Naing, S. S., & Chaikittiporn, C. (2010). Prevalence and risk factors of low back pain among Thai and Myanmar migrant seafood processing factory workers in Samut Sakorn Province, Thailand. *Industrial Health, 48 (3) 283-291.*

Tortora, G., & Grabowski, S. (2003). Principals of anatomy and physiology (10 e éd.). *New York: John Wiley et Sons Inc.*

Troup, J. D. G. (1996). Back pain and epidemiology review: The epidemiology and cost of back pain: Clinical Standards Advisory Group (Committee Chaired by Michael Rosen). Her Majesty's Stationery Office, London, 1994.(Respectively 89pp. and 72pp. paperback,£ 14.00: ISBN 0-11-321887-7 and ISBN 0-11-321889-3). *Social Science & Medicine, 42(4), 561–563.*

Turk, D. C., Meichenbaum, D., & Genest, M. (1983). *Pain and behavioral medicine: A cognitive-behavioral perspective (Vol. 1). Guilford Press.*

van der Velde, G., & Mierau, D. (2000). The effect of exercise on percentile rank aerobic capacity, pain, and self-rated disability in patients with chronic low-back pain: a retrospective chart review. *Archives of Physical Medicine and Rehabilitation, 81(11), 1457–1463.*

Van Hall, G., Raaymakers, J. S., Saris, W. H., & Wagenmakers, A. J. (1995). Ingestion of branched-chain amino acids and tryptophan during sustained exercise in man: failure to affect performance. *The Journal of Physiology, 486(3), 789–794.*

van Tulder, M. W., Koes, B. W., & Bouter, L. M. (1995). A cost-of-illness study of back pain in The Netherlands. *Pain, 62(2), 233–240.*

Van Tulder, M. W., Koes, B. W., & Bouter, L. M. (1997). Conservative treatment of acute and chronic nonspecific low back pain: a systematic review of randomized controlled trials of the most common interventions. *Spine, 22 (18) 2128-2156.*

Van Tulder, M. W., Malmivaara, A., Esmail, R., & Koes, B. W. (1999). Exercise therapy for low back pain. *The Cochrane database of systematic reviews, (2), CD000335-CD000335.*

Van Tulder, M., Becker, A., Bekkering, T., Breen, A., Gil del Real, M. T., Hutchinson, A., ... Malmivaara, A. (2006). Chapter 3 European guidelines for the management of acute nonspecific low back pain in primary care. *European Spine Journal, 15, s169–s191.*

Van Tulder, M., Furlan, A., Bombardier, C., Bouter, L., & Group, E. B. of the C. C. B. R. (2003). Updated method guidelines for systematic reviews in the cochrane collaboration back review group. *Spine, 28(12), 1290–1299.*

Vinjamuri, R., Mao, Z.-H., Sclabassi, R., & Sun, M. (2006). Limitations of surface EMG signals of extrinsic muscles in predicting postures of human hand. In Engineering in Medicine and Biology Society, 2006. EMBS'06. *28th Annual International Conference of the IEEE (pp. 5491–5494). IEEE.*

Waddell, G., & Burton, A. K. (2001). Occupational health guidelines for the management of low back pain at work: evidence review. *Occupational Medicine, 51(2), 124–135.*

Waddell, G., Feder, G., & Lewis, M. (1997). Systematic reviews of bed rest and advice to stay active for acute low back pain. *Br J Gen Pract, 47 (423) 647-652.*

Waddell, G., Somerville, D., Henderson, I., & Newton, M. (1992). Objective clinical evaluation of physical impairment in chronic low back pain. *Spine, 17(6), 617–628.*

Walker, A., & Cooper, I. (2000). *Adult dental health survey: oral health in the United Kingdom 1998. Stationery Office.*

Walker, B. F. (2000). The prevalence of low back pain: a systematic review of the literature from 1966 to 1998. *Clinical Spine Surgery, 13(3), 205–217.*

Watson, K. D., Papageorgiou, A. C., Jones, G. T., Taylor, S., Symmons, D. P., Silman, A. J., & Macfarlane, G. J. (2002). Low back pain in schoolchildren: occurrence and characteristics. *Pain, 97 (1) 87-92.*

Watson, K. D., Papageorgiou, A. C., Jones, G. T., Taylor, S., Symmons, D. P. M., Silman, A. J., & Macfarlane, G. J. (2003). Low back pain in schoolchildren: the role of mechanical and psychosocial factors. *Archives of Disease in Childhood, 88(1), 12–17.*

Weiss, L., Dowling, D. J., Domingo, R. A., Schaefer, L. A., Salomon, V., Flynn, E., ... Pobre, T. (2010). Rehabilitation issues. *Physical Medicine and Rehabilitation, 401.*

WHITE III, A. A., & Gordon, S. L. (1982). Synopsis: workshop on idiopathic low-back pain. *Spine, 7(2), 141–149.*

Wijnhoven, H. A., de Vet, H. C., Smit, H. A., & Picavet, H. S. J. (2006). Hormonal and reproductive factors are associated with chronic low back pain and chronic upper extremity pain in women–the MORGEN study. *Spine, 31(13), 1496-1502.*

Wilder, D. G., Aleksiev, A. R., Magnusson, M. L., Pope, M. H., Spratt, K. F., & Goel, V. K. (1996). Muscular response to sudden load: a tool to evaluate fatigue and rehabilitation. *Spine, 21 (22) 2628-2639.*

Wilke, H.-J., Wolf, S., Claes, L. E., Arand, M., & Wiesend, A. (1995). Stability Increase of the Lumbar Spine With Different Muscle Groups: A Biomechanical In Vitro Study. *Spine, 20(2), 192–197.*

Williams, P. C. (1955). Examination and conservative treatment for disk lesions of the lower spine. *Clinical Orthopaedics, 5, 28-40.*

wk Lee, S., & Kim, S. Y. (2015). Effects of hip exercises for chronic low-back pain patients with lumbar instability. *Journal of Physical Therapy Science, 27(2), 345–348.*

Youdas, J. W., Guck, B. R., Hebrink, R. C., Rugotzke, J. D., Madson, T. J., & Hollman, J. H. (2008). An electromyographic analysis of the Ab-Slide exercise, abdominal crunch, supine double leg thrust, and side bridge in healthy young adults: implications for rehabilitation professionals. *The Journal of Strength & Conditioning Research, 22 (6) 1939-1946.*

Zipp, P. (1982). Recommendations for the standardization of lead positions in surface electromyography. *European Journal of Applied Physiology and Occupational Physiology, 50(1), 41–54.*

Printed in the United States
By Bookmasters